20512

WHEN CANCER COMES

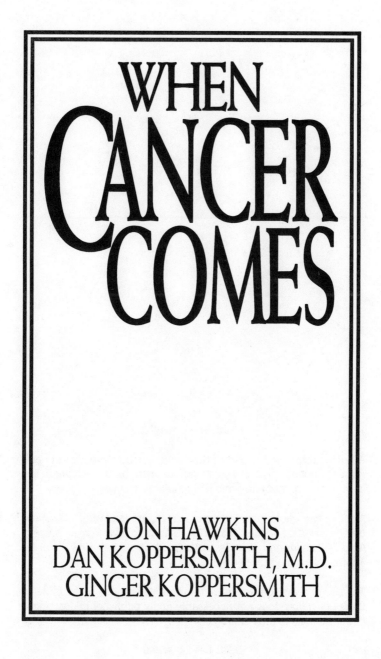

WHEN CANCER COMES

DON HAWKINS
DAN KOPPERSMITH, M.D.
GINGER KOPPERSMITH

MOODY PRESS

CHICAGO

*To the loving memory of Dr. Jim Mahoney,
our friend and colleague of many years at Rapha,
whose wholehearted love for God
and unconditional love for people
was evident to all with whom he came in contact,
and who has now moved from the pain
of a prolonged battle with cancer of the pancreas
to the delight of a pain-free eternity
in the presence of the Lord he loved*

CONTENTS

Preface		9
Acknowledgments		11
1.	A War Story	13
2.	What Is Cancer?	25
3.	A Perspective on Physical Illness	43
4.	How Do You Get Cancer?	63
5.	Cancer and the Physical	87
6.	Cancer and the Emotional	105
7.	Cancer and the Spiritual	127
8.	Treating Cancer	149
9.	Encouraging the Cancer Patient's Family	173
10.	Living with Cancer, Dying of Cancer	199
11.	Preventing Cancer	227
12.	Research Toward Eliminating Cancer	247
	Notes	267
	Glossary	271

PREFACE

Not everyone who reads a book asks why the author wrote it. But for many people, the answer to that question sheds light on the subject of the book itself.

As we prepared to write this book, we discovered that most books about cancer fall into one of two categories: clinical discussions covering the wealth of data about various forms of cancer and cancer treatments, or first-person accounts of battles with cancer of one kind or another.

Our purpose in *this* book was to approach the issue from a different perspective. Convinced that God is concerned about our whole selves, "spirit, soul, and body" (1 Thessalonians 5:23), we sought to address cancer, which we perceived to be a major concern of people from all walks of life, from a spiritual, emotional, and physical perspective.

For Dr. Dan Koppersmith, one of several strong motivating factors was the tragedy of losing his father to cancer during Dan's infant years. Another is the personal satisfaction of Dan's psychiatric practice. Working on the Rapha Christian inpatient treatment program in Houston and in an outpatient practice, Dan often helps patients and their families deal with issues related to cancer. He has discovered that appropriate therapy can help heal the intense emotional trauma surrounding cancer and that a strong personal faith enables the patient to accept what cannot be changed and work at changing what can be. Sharing how the combination of therapy and personal faith has helped him and others is part of Dan's motivation in writing this book.

For many years, Ginger Koppersmith has worked directly with cancer patients and those who treat them at the University of Texas Health Science Center, at the Houston School of Nursing, and at the M.D. Anderson Cancer Center. However, a stronger personal motivating factor has been Ginger's close friendship with Angela, whom she met during her research at M.D. Anderson. (Angela's story is told in chapter 4.) The two women challenged each other spiritually, emotionally, and intellectually, developing a friendship that far exceeded the usual patient-health care professional relationship. Seeing the devastation produced by cancer in the life of this close friend, and having learned the importance of a balanced approach to the spiritual, emotional, and physical/medical issues brought about by cancer, Ginger was eager to help with *When Cancer Comes.*

For nineteen years Don pastored churches, then became involved in radio counseling ministries. Frequently he found his ministry directed toward those who suffered from the effects of cancer and toward their families. His own family experienced widely the effects of cancer. Eight of his father's brothers and sisters were diagnosed with cancer—ironically all from different forms of the disease—and six died. They are mentioned in chapter 1, and their stories are told in chapter 11.

The three authors, believing there to be a need for a Christian book to comprehensively address the wide range of issues precipitated by cancer, seeing the emotional pain and spiritual struggles precipitated by cancer, and concerned by the devastation produced in the lives of many who sought help from so-called alternative therapies that proved to be dead-ends, have sought to give a balanced medical, emotional, and spiritual perspective for when cancer comes.

ACKNOWLEDGMENTS

Special thanks to Kathy Hawkins, who provided significant encouragement, as well as insight, throughout this project.

To the many individuals who were willing to share their stories to give others insight, encouragement, and hope—Angela, Candy and Lee, Liz and Bill, Ron, Dianna and Jessica, Judith and Stephane, Cliff and Gloria, Shannon and all Jim's friends from Rapha, Casey, Andrea, and all Debbie's friends from Lake Pointe, Jim and Juanita, Betty and Robert and the rest of the "clan," and Phyllis, and to all the family, friends, and treatment team members who served each of them.

To Ruth Anne Franks for tireless labor under difficult circumstances, typing and retyping the manuscript and revisions.

To the "Life Perspectives" team—including Jerry Bostick, Paul Klassen, Don Sapaugh, Pam Moize, and to Becky Daniel and Thom Justice, and Cecil Price.

To the Moody Press team—notably to Joseph O'Day for his work in shaping the concept, to Jim Bell for his vision to bring it to reality, and to Ella Lindvall and the rest of the editorial, production, and publicity team.

Last, but not least, to Heath, Brent, Karen, and Donna, and to Chris, Albert, and Karissa for extra special encouragement.

Most of all, thanks to the God whose grace has been sufficient for the project, and whose provision provides the ultimate answer for cancer.

1

A WAR STORY

Tom thought there was no possible way he could have cancer. He just would not allow it.

After removing his size fifty jacket, he squeezed his two-hundred-twenty-plus pounds into a chair and crossed his size thirteen cowboy boots in the small conference room of one of the physicians at M.D. Anderson Hospital. Tom had come face to face with reality—prostate cancer. He was going to have to start confronting something he didn't want to face.

Tom had found himself in many a scrape over the course of his life, during which time he rose from the oil fields of West Texas as a roughneck to his present position as president of a Houston-based oil and gas company. But this was something different.

"Come on, Doc," Tom countered in his gravelly voice, "so I've got cancer. This is the best place in the world to get treated for cancer. Can't you just zap me with some of that radiation stuff, give me a few pills to take, and turn me loose? After all, cancer schmancer. All them cancers are pretty much the same."

Dr. Blake* smiled as he shook his head. "Tom, I'm afraid it's not that simple. You see, you've been telling me that you've

---

* Certain names, descriptive elements, and other details in this book have been changed for purposes of confidentiality.

been having this trouble going to the bathroom for over a year now—that sometimes it actually takes you as long as an hour to urinate."

"Well, Doc, that's not the whole story. I mean, it's like, with the phones ringing and all those interruptions, the bathroom is just the best place to read through contracts and stuff."

Though more slightly built than Tom, Dr. Blake did not back off. "C'mon, Tom. Are you trying to tell me you don't have that kind of trouble urinating—that it doesn't take you that long?"

The rugged oilman leaned back in his chair, causing it to groan noticeably. Throwing his hands up in the air, he said, "OK, Doc. You win. I've got a problem. After all, it's only been that way for about a year. So you should be able to take care of it pretty easily, right?"

"Not so fast, Tom. You see, most cancers start growing pretty slowly. It may actually take a cancer ten, twenty, even forty years to grow. If you catch those cancers during the early stages, before they've grown big enough to do serious damage, they're almost always curable—in fact, our researchers tell me that three-fourths of all cancers could be cured if people would just practice self-examination or get regular checkups."

Tom interrupted rather brusquely. "OK, Doc, I hear what you're saying. I didn't go to the doctor soon enough. I confess, I just didn't have time. But who does? Besides, if I spent all my time running back and forth to the doctor, the people I work with would consider me a wimp."

Dr. Blake chuckled. "This is certainly not the first time I've heard that thinking, Tom. But facts are facts: One out of three people in this country will be diagnosed with some kind of cancer in their lifetime. That means that three out of every four families will have someone come down with cancer. In fact, a friend of mine, who grew up in Birmingham, Alabama, when the steel mills were in operation, came from a family of twelve kids. So far, my friend Jimmy is one of only two members of that family not to develop cancer of some kind. Twelve kids in his family! Two died when they were babies. But every single one who lived to be an adult, except Jimmy and his sister, developed cancer of some kind—lung cancer, liver cancer, pancreatic cancer, prostate cancer, breast cancer—they had it all. In fact, cancer has killed most of Jimmy's brothers and sisters."

"So how did he survive?" Tom asked.

"Well, he goes go to the doctor every six months for a checkup, but I don't think you'd call him a wimp. He's not as big as you are, but he's a pretty rugged guy. He was a marine— fought in World War II—then he spent over forty years working on the railroad. Started off shoveling coal as a fireman before he became a long-haul engineer."

"Hogheads, that's what they call them." Tom grinned. "One of my best friends spent many a year on the business end of a Southern Pacific locomotive. Mostly freight, but a few passengers—even ran the 'Sunset Limited' for a while. But let's get back to me, Doc. You told me I've got cancer. But cut to the chase. Am I going to make it? Or is this thing going to kill me?"

Cancer isn't a death sentence; it's just an illness.

"To be honest with you, Tom, I can't say for sure. We've nailed down your diagnosis—cancer of the prostate. But we're still working on your prognosis."

"Diagnosis, prognosis . . . you guys use these fancy words. I never did graduate from high school. Spit it out in plain English, Doc."

"It's really pretty simple, Tom. *Diagnosis* is just a big word for pinpointing exactly what kind of cancer you have. After all, cancer is not just a single disease—it's a group of diseases. Some people say that medical researchers have identified more than a hundred different types of cancer.

"Now all cancers have certain things in common—body cells growing out of control—and they can spread, or metastasize—that's another one of our fancy words—through the blood or lymph nodes to other parts of the body."

"Y' mean, this cancer down in my prostate could actually go straight to my brain?"

The doctor smiled again. "Well, that's not likely to happen, Tom. But I did see a man in here just yesterday who had colon cancer that spread to his liver. That's a bad situation. Right now he's at pretty serious risk as far as making it."

Noticing the unease of the rugged oilman sitting across from him, Dr. Blake hastened to add, "You need to remember, Tom. Cancer isn't a death sentence; it's just an illness. Our statistics indicate that nearly half the people diagnosed with cancer will be alive five years after their diagnosis."

"Alive, sure, but how?" Tom countered, a scowl on his leathery face. "Living like some kind of vegetable, hooked up to those machines that feed and water patients in some kind of intensive care?"

"Not really. In fact, most cancers that aren't really curable can be treated in such a way that the patient can have a relatively normal life. Sort of like someone with diabetes. Do you know anyone who's a diabetic?"

"My brother. He was always the studious type, a bookworm. He's three years older than me. He has to take a shot every day, watch what he eats, and all that."

"But he lives a fairly normal life, wouldn't you say?"

"Yeah, I suppose you could say that. But he doesn't have as much fun as me! Because he's never worked in the oil fields. We work hard and play hard—eat and drink pretty much what we want to."

"Well, you and I will be talking about that, plus a lot more, next time we get together. I want to see you in here early next week—check with my receptionist for a specific appointment. By that time we'll try to have your prognosis figured out. I wouldn't get antsy about that—even though it's another twenty-five-cent term. A *prognosis* is just a prediction of how you're going to do. It's sort of an educated guess based on statistics of other cases. Nobody—not even somebody with the gift of prophecy—will know exactly how you're going to do. But we'll try to give you a pretty good idea of what to expect, based on your type of cancer and how far advanced the tests show it to be. Your physical fitness is a plus. After all, you're a pretty rugged guy. But we'll look at any medical conditions that show up in your examinations. I'm sure you've been to the doctor a few times."

"So the prognosis will tell me how I'm gonna do?"

"Generally," Dr. Blake responded, "but not precisely. Actually, there are many people who beat the odds. I remember Richard Block, chairman of the board of H&R Block. He came down here to M.D. Anderson from Kansas City several years ago. The odds against his surviving were about a million to one —that's a million to one *against.* He had the worst case of lung cancer you could imagine—he smoked heavily. I remember our senior doctors telling him 'Surgery, radiation, chemotherapy— you're going to be one sick boy. But that's the only way we have any chance of making you well.'"

Ninety percent of those surveyed picked cancer as the one thing they feared the most.

"So he beat the odds." The intent look on Tom's seamed countenance indicated the anxiety he felt about his own condition.

Dr. Blake's smile grew even larger. "He sure did. Five years later the man was cancer free—he even plays tennis regularly now. So it can be beaten. But a lot of it is up to you—your personal faith, your will to live, and, of course, your getting good medical care. But I'm not going to kid you, Tom. It's going to be combat . . . armed combat."*

Armed Combat

When Cancer Comes is designed to arm you with information and insight, encouragement and motivation, so that you will be able to succeed in combating cancer. It may be that you have cancer yourself. Perhaps you've just found out, or maybe you've known for some time now. Or perhaps you're seriously at risk for cancer. Like Dr. Blake's friend, Jimmy, you may have grown up in a city where just breathing the air was the equivalent of smoking many packs of cigarettes a day. Or you may have been a DES baby, significantly at risk for the kinds of cancer that frequently affect females whose mothers used that medication. Perhaps a relative, a close friend, or a loved one has cancer, or is at risk. Whatever the case, the chances are that, to some degree or another, cancer is one of your major concerns.

A few years ago, an extensive public opinion poll posed the question, "What do you fear most?"[1] A list of possible an-

---

* See chapter 4 for the rest of Tom's story.

swers included all forms of calamities and maladies ranging from earthquakes and atomic war to heart attacks and cancer. Ninety percent of those surveyed picked cancer as the one thing they feared the most.

In Dr. Koppersmith's work with Rapha Treatment Center, treating individuals who are depressed or suffering anxiety disorders, the fear of cancer ranks as one of his patients' major concerns. He has observed that the threat of cancer produces two major emotional effects (discussed in-depth in chapter 6). The first is *fear*, an intense emotion of dread that focuses on a specific object—in this case the possibility of a disease that will be disabling, produce intense pain, and ultimately lead to an untimely death. The second major emotion produced by cancer is *depression.* As Tom was about to discover, and as Liz, Debbie, Cliff, and the other individuals whose cases we will follow in this book would find out, people whose lives are touched by cancer are just not the same. They suffer loss. And loss produces anger. Anger, focused inward, leads to depression.

Frequently there is a strong spiritual component to this depression (discussed in-depth in chapter 7). Even those whose lives are undergirded by strong Christian faith often raise the questions, "Why me? Do I deserve this? Why did God allow me to come down with cancer?"

Most health professionals consider cancer to be catastrophic. Our experiences—as a medical doctor, as a nurse/researcher, and as a pastor—have convinced us of the catastrophic nature of cancer. That's one reason we felt compelled to write *When Cancer Comes*—to help those who are facing cancer, not to deny or minimize the incredible toll cancer takes on those who have it and on their families. In addition to the major cases we will pursue throughout this book, we will frequently reference others from our years of clinical and pastoral experience in order to show cancer's devastating impact.

A Positive Purpose

But our purpose is not simply to convince you of the catastrophic nature of cancer. Rather, we have written to motivate you, to strengthen your faith, to bolster your resolve—in short, to convince you that cancer is treatable, its risks beatable.

There *is* hope for the person who has been diagnosed with cancer! Our goal in writing is to provide the cancer patient, and all those impacted by cancer, with the ultimate emotional and spiritual antidote—*hope!*

Right now you may be thinking, *But isn't a lot of cancer terminal?* Certainly, no question. But a lot of cancer is not. The issue is not whether cancer is terminal. Life itself is terminal. After all, a wise leader from biblical days once pointed out that every single individual has an appointment with death (Hebrews 9:27). The only question for each of us is, "When?"

Our experience has shown us that a person's attitude about life in general, and cancer in particular, plays a key role in how he or she responds to the disease. If a person feels hopeless, it's almost as if the cancer becomes incurable—even with the best of medical care. On the other hand, for the person who combines strong personal faith with a positive fighting attitude and the best medical care available, the chances of beating cancer are much better.

Serious illnesses such as cancer produce questions, questions that are not always easy to ask a physician, though we each encourage cancer patients with whom we have contact to raise those questions. *When Cancer Comes* is designed to help provide answers to many of these. Most of the questions, and their answers, are found in easy-to-follow dialogue between patients like Tom and medical and pastoral caregivers, supportive family members, and friends.

For some questions there are no simple answers:

"Why am I experiencing this?"
"What will happen to my family—and to me—if I don't get better?"
"Do my doctors really know what they're doing?"
"Why me? Why not someone else?"
"Even if I do beat this illness, what about my sexual desires and my quality of life?"
"Where is God in all of this?"
"Will I be able to stand the pain?"

Then there's the question of cost. "Won't having cancer destroy me financially?"

A Financial Drain

There's no question that cancer creates a major expense—both for those who have it and for society in general. According to a national center for health statistics study,[2] cancer accounts for about 10 percent of the total cost of disease in the United States. According to the study, the overall cost of cancer in 1985 was more than $71 billion, including nearly $22 billion in direct medical costs. Additional expenses included the loss of productivity, plus costs related to premature death. Certainly Tom was about to confront serious economic and personal costs in ways he couldn't even imagine as he sat in Dr. Blake's office.

For Tom, and for the other cases we will pursue, there would be emotional costs as well, such as anxiety, reduced self-esteem, and even strong feelings of guilt: *God must be judging me for something terrible I did*, or, *If only I'd never smoked*, or, *If only I had stopped eating so much fat in my diet perhaps this wouldn't have happened.*

We recognize the reality of legitimate guilt and the importance of dealing with it. And we cannot deny the existence of consequences for certain behaviors. That's the way our wise Creator designed the universe. For example, one of man's longtime dreams has been to fly. Unfortunately, history is littered with individuals who sought to defy the law of gravity and suffered the consequences of their defiance. So it is with factors such as smoking and diet, generally identified as major environmental contributors. They frequently cause cancer-related consequences.

However, we often encourage those we talk to about cancer to face the difference between legitimate guilt and false guilt. It's important to recognize that God can forgive us, and we must forgive ourselves. Frequently this takes time and counsel. What we urge individuals to do is to first forgive themselves, then stop focusing on the past with its "What ifs" and "If onlys." Instead, we encourage those who are combating cancer to focus on the present, on the task at hand.

Nolan Ryan has been recognized as one of the most successful professional baseball players of all time. Any man who could go out on a given night and pitch a no-hitter against men twenty years his junior—men who in many cases weren't even born when he began his major league career—must have a phenomenal ability to focus on the task at hand.

Recently, after he experienced one of his worst outings— giving up six runs and walking seven batters in an ineffective five inning stint—Ryan was asked if such a poor performance would affect his continued desire to play or prompt him to consider taking the retirement route of most professional athletes his age. "Not at all," the veteran replied. "That game is history now."

More and earlier screening for cancer, plus adoption of a high-fiber, low-fat diet by all Americans, could save between 30,000 and 150,000 lives each year.

In other words, whether he pitches a no-hitter the previous outing or bombs, Nolan Ryan's approach is always the same: he gets up the next day, carries out his extensive regimen of workouts, and prepares himself scrupulously for his next turn to pitch. That's precisely the approach we advocate in *When Cancer Comes.* We focus on hard work in the present, plus an active faith for the future.

Why Can't We Prevent Cancer?

But perhaps you're thinking, with all of our marvelous technological strides, why haven't we been able to wipe out cancer? Why can't we just *prevent* it? After all, earlier this century tuberculosis was the most feared disease, and smallpox and the plague before that. We've pretty much taken care of them. That success occurred, however, because these diseases have specific, known causes, such as bacteria and viruses.

The National Cancer Institute has announced a public goal of reducing cancer mortality by 50 percent by the year 2000. They suggest that more and earlier screening for cancer, plus adoption of a high-fiber, low-fat diet by all Americans, could save between 30,000 and 150,000 lives each year.

But maybe prevention is no longer an issue for you or someone close to you. Like Tom, you may have been given that feared diagnosis. How quickly do you need to get started with treatment? Right now is the best time to begin treating your cancer. Some forms of cancer grow extremely slowly. Others grow amazingly fast. Still others develop slowly, but, by the time they are diagnosed, the sheer magnitude of the billions of cancer cells present means that time is of the essence.

When Dr. Blake told Tom the story about Richard Block, he didn't include the details that we learned firsthand in an extended interview with the cofounder of one of the world's most famous tax preparation companies. It was a sunny afternoon one April 15, in the garden outside Mr. Block's mansion in South Kansas City. But the subject of discussion that day had nothing to do with income taxes. Instead, Richard Block was relating the story of his mortal combat with lung cancer.

"My doctors put me in touch with M.D. Anderson Hospital, and the staff there didn't give me any choice. I told them that I planned to fly down to spend a weekend at our beach house, then show up at M.D. Anderson first thing Monday morning. This was on a Friday.

"The doctor told me, 'Mr. Block, if you're planning on waiting until Monday, don't bother to come. It's that serious. You need to be on the next plane to Houston. We want you in here tonight. Based on the X rays and records we've seen, we'll be starting treatment first thing in the morning.'"

Mr. Block, wearing a white tennis shirt and shorts, paused to take a sip from his glass of lemonade. "I remember what the doctor told me next like it was yesterday. He said, 'Mr. Block, we're going to make you one sick boy. But it's your only chance to get well.'"

Perhaps you have known for some time that you are at risk for cancer. Or maybe you know you have it but you're still wrestling with denial, struggling to face the necessity for treatment. We hope this book underscores for you the urgency of joining the combat, of getting the help you need.

And, no, your life will never be quite the way it was before. But remember, this is not the only change you've ever faced. In fact, everything in life involves change. And, yes, change is stressful. But you've dealt successfully with change before. When you were a child, you learned to walk and talk. Then you went off to school, and that meant giving up spending all that time at home. Learning to drive, getting married, having children—these bring about changes, responsibilities, limitations. Most roads are built with curves—some sharp, some gentle, some not so gentle. What you are doing right now is just rounding one of the sharper curves in your life.

But keep going! There is hope. There are options for you ahead. If you have cancer, or if someone close to you does, the option of not having cancer no longer exists. But there are other viable options—treatment options—and, most important of all, the option to do what Tom, Liz, Phyllis, Cliff, and others did—the option to fight back, the option of securing the best medical care.

We have written *When Cancer Comes* to have an impact on three areas of your life:

1 *Physically,* we want you to seek the best possible medical care and to devote your own best efforts and resources to fighting cancer. We want you to become convinced that cancer *can* be beaten. A cancer diagnosis *isn't* an automatic death sentence. But it must be taken seriously and fought vigorously.

2 *Emotionally,* our goal is to help you avoid the danger of denial, or of stuffing or repressing your feelings of anger about the disease and its impact on your life. Several years after his cancer diagnosis, on a warm June day less than two months after our conversation with Richard Block, a crowd of more than eight hundred gathered at Barney Allis Plaza in downtown Kansas City to hear Mr. Block and Amanda Blake, star of early television's "Gunsmoke," talk about their personal battles with cancer. Other cancer patients shared the podium during the two-hour "Celebration of Life."

Mrs. Blake, who successfully fought mouth cancer, talked about her attitude as "one of the undefeated." Following the rally, she agreed with Mr. Block's assessment that "the real fight against cancer is getting in your mind that, if you do everything possible, you have every chance of beating it." Mr. Block cited medical evidence that patients who learn to express and process their emotions, including anger, instead of simply adopting a stoic attitude, have a better chance of coping with the disease.

Our experience has shown us the validity of Mr. Block's assertion. This book has been written to encourage the proper expression of emotions and to show you how.

3 But the heart of our purpose in writing *When Cancer Comes* is *spiritual.* We are convinced that the most important dimension in this battle involves a personal trust in the Creator, who made our bodies, whose sovereign hand guides the universe, and who has provided through His Son the ultimate answer for a dilemma even more serious than cancer or any physical disease—the sin that infects each of us.

That's why the ultimate treatment option the three of us would like to personally encourage you to exercise immediately is the option of confident, optimistic faith in Christ—faith for forgiveness and a personal relationship with Him, and faith for each day, each hour, to face whatever comes, including cancer.

2

WHAT IS CANCER?

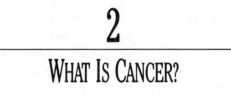

U nlike Tom, who had been oblivious to the threat of cancer prior to his diagnosis, Liz had lived for years with the fear that cancer would somehow invade her life. Twenty-four years earlier, Liz had lost her father to stomach cancer. Then less than a year before she called our nationwide talk show, her mother had been diagnosed with stomach cancer.

As Liz explained, "It was a time of great stress in our family—high anxiety. I've been afraid I'd get cancer for a long time. In fact, it's almost as though I had a premonition I would die of cancer. For the past several months I've had this persistent cough. Then the other morning I found myself coughing up blood. I'm really glad you're doing a program on this topic."

When asked by Dr. Koppersmith about her emotional state, Liz responded in a quiet voice: "I'm scared to death." Such a strong emotional reaction toward cancer is normal. Dr. Donald Nichols suggests that every cancer patient goes through the same stages of grief as those identified by Elizabeth Kubler-Ross in her work with death and dying.[1] Liz's initial response, as might be expected, was denial. Despite recognizing that her symptoms were growing more serious, she had postponed scheduling a checkup, hoping that the problem would somehow lessen and go away. But it didn't.

Now it was time for Liz, goaded by the encouragement of Dr. Koppersmith, to take action. The next day, hands shaking, she dialed her physician's office to schedule an appointment. The following afternoon she found herself seated in his waiting room, hands clenched together in her lap, nervously waiting. *Dear God, don't let it be,* she prayed silently. *Let it be something else—a persistent cold, allergies, anything but cancer.*

After all, Liz was living the good life. She, her husband, their two teenaged children, and their dog were enjoying the ideal middle-class experience. Their two-story, three-bedroom, brick home was an island of happiness, the center of a comfortable life. Despite her concerns over her mother, Liz had remained active in church work, volunteered to be part of her local political action committee, and even participated in a recent "life chain" to demonstrate her concern about abortion. She and her husband, both of whom had trusted Christ at an early age, had introduced their young children to faith and had taken them to church regularly.

Liz found her troubled thoughts interrupted by a receptionist calling her name. When kindly Dr. Franklin and his nurse entered her treatment room, she found herself minimizing the problem. "I have a bit of a cough—I just can't seem to shake it. But I'm sure it's not anything serious."

But under Dr. Franklin's gentle yet persistent questioning, Liz finally admitted that the cough had been worsening for months and that there had been times when she actually coughed up blood. "I'm really scared, Dr. Franklin. My father died of cancer. My mother has it now. But my symptoms aren't anything like what *they* went through."

After a careful physical examination, including a chest X ray and a sputum test, the nurse suggested that Liz stop by the receptionist's desk to schedule another appointment, preferably within forty-eight hours. "That soon?" Liz wasn't sure she could spare the time. "I shifted several things from today until later in the week so that I could come in today."

"Dr. Franklin insists," the nurse replied gently but firmly. "I think he'll want to go over the results of today's tests with you."

Two days later the same nurse ushered Liz into Dr. Franklin's cluttered yet comfortable office. Books and medical journals were scattered across his desk, while crowded bookshelves lined two walls. Late afternoon sunshine streamed through partially open Venetian blinds. Dust motes floated on unseen air currents across the rays of sunlight. Finally, after what seemed an eternity—it was actually only a couple of minutes—Dr. Franklin entered the room.

"Liz, I'm afraid the news isn't good. The X rays show a small but definite mass on your left lung. And even though sputum cytology isn't always accepted as definite, your sputum test indicated the presence of malignant cells. You ought to have a CAT scan, to confirm what I suspect. And I'm sending you immediately to Dr. Morris over at the oncology clinic. He's a specialist in this sort of thing. Oncologists are specially trained doctors who deal with cancer and cancer patients."

Liz raised her hand in protest. "But, Dr. Franklin, why can't I just see you? After all, you've been our family doctor for twenty years now."

Gently overriding the protest of his obviously anxious patient, Dr. Franklin picked up the telephone at his desk and punched in the number for his receptionist. "Can we delay my next couple of patients? I really need to take some time to explain this situation to Liz." He paused for a moment, then smiled as he gripped the telephone receiver. "A cancellation? Why, that's excellent. In fact, I'd call it providential."

Replacing the receiver, Dr. Franklin leaned back in his chair. "All right, Liz. I was your dad's doctor. I've been your mom's primary physician, and yours as well. I've been seeing you since you were a little girl in pigtails missing your two front teeth. So I feel I should take the time to tell you more about what cancer is and, more important, what you can do about it."

Leaning forward in his chair, Dr. Franklin picked up a brochure from atop the stack of papers on the left side of his desk. "The timing on this is remarkable, Liz. Just last week I attended a cancer briefing for general practice physicians. So a lot of the facts about cancer are fresh in my mind. Perhaps I can give you some information that will encourage you, some insight to help you prepare for the battle ahead. And Liz, you *do* have a battle ahead."

Liz felt tears welling up in her eyes as she attempted to express her thanks.

"There's a lot more to learn than I can share with you

today. And I can tell you right now, Liz—you'll find out a great deal from Dr. Morris, especially about treatment options and what may be most appropriate for you."

"Not surgery, I hope," Liz interrupted. "I'm just not sure I could handle it again. Remember how sick I was for so long after my gallbladder was removed?"

As Dr. Franklin smiled again, Liz noticed the wrinkles in his face and the crinkles at the corners of his eyes. "I'm sure there'll be no surgery unless it's absolutely necessary, Liz. But I can't guarantee there won't be. There are thirteen different kinds of lung cancers, but several of the most common kinds are best treated with surgery—*if* they are caught before they spread beyond the lung. One kind, often referred to as *oat-cell*, isn't treated with surgery. But I want to assure you that if surgery is necessary Dr. Morris will recommend an excellent thoracic surgeon who is experienced at this sort of thing—and only if it's the best way to save your life."

Lung cancer is one of the most lethal of the more than one hundred forms cancer takes.

Without thinking, the nervous woman interrupted the physician again. "But why did this have to happen, doctor? I mean, why me?" Catching herself, Liz apologized for interrupting. "It's just that I can't believe this has happened to me. Did I inherit this? Did I do something wrong? Is God punishing me? And why, *lung* cancer? I don't smoke . . . never have. Dad smoked, but he didn't even get lung cancer."

Although he didn't say so to Liz, Dr. Franklin remembered the words of the cancer specialist he had heard at the physician's briefing the previous week: "Lung cancer is one of the most lethal of the more than one hundred forms cancer takes." A frown creased his face as he remembered hearing that lung cancer was now the leading cause of death by cancer in both men and women, supplanting breast cancer among women. He recalled the chart he had seen—more than 143,000 lung cancer deaths in America in 1991, with more than 300,000 annual deaths anticipated by the turn of the century.

Dr. Franklin also remembered clearly the words of the re-search oncologist: "The number one cause is smoking. And passive smoking—exposure to tobacco smoke from relatives, friends, or workers—is a serious factor in causing lung cancer among those who don't smoke. The Environmental Protection Agency estimates that between 500 and 5,000 cases of lung can-cer are diagnosed each year in nonsmokers as a result of them inhaling someone else's smoke."

"Let's start with some basics, Liz," he began. "First of all, you probably think of cancer as a single disease. It really isn't. In fact, there are more than a hundred different kinds of cancer. Lung cancer, for example, is quite different from stomach can-cer. Skin cancer is different from bone cancer. Leukemia is dif-ferent from breast cancer."

"Maybe that's why it's so hard for them to find a cure," Liz responded, hope mingling with fear on her face.

"I'd have to agree. In fact, at the symposium last week, they didn't say a lot about cures for cancers. But I did learn that close to 90 percent of all cancers can be prevented, and many forms of cancer can be cured."

Shifting in her seat, Liz listened attentively as Dr. Franklin continued. "Back in 1913 when the American Cancer Society was first founded, most people considered cancer a sort of death sentence. In fact, during the 1930s, less than 20 percent of cancer patients were still alive five years after their initial treatment.[2] But we've seen a lot of improvement since then. By the 1970s, over 30 percent of cancer patients were pronouned 'cured' after five years. As of a couple of years ago, the number was up to 50 percent.

"Now, of course, some cancers can be considered cured much more quickly than others. For example, the doctor I heard speak suggested that he and others frequently do not consider breast cancer to be cured after five years—there's still a serious chance of recurrence. On the other hand, childhood leukemia can be considered cured just three years following treatment."

"Does that mean there's less cancer today?" Liz asked.

The doctor shook his head. "No. In fact, the number of cancers is increasing in the United States. And the major culprit is smoking. We've certainly made rapid strides in treating cancers, and we've done a better job with the surgeon general's warnings about the dangers of smoking. But the total number of new cancer cases is still increasing. Statistics indicate that one out of three people in the United States will be diagnosed with cancer at some time during the course of their lives."

Liz felt a shudder run through her body as she thought about her two children. Her mathematically attuned mind wrestled with numbers, and she came to a grim conclusion: "I guess that means cancer will affect three-fourths of all the families in the United States."

Dr. Franklin nodded. "It's a pretty frightening statistic, isn't it? But the good news I heard last week is that 75 percent of all cancer could be cured—if only everyone would practice prevention, self-examination, and regular checkups."

Blushing with shame, Liz thought about how long she had waited to check into the reason for her persistent cough. "I guess I should have come in a couple months ago. It was so dumb of me to wait. But I guess I'm like a lot of other people. I just don't like to think about what you doctors may find."

A kind expression spread across Dr. Franklin's face. "Now don't be so hard on yourself, Liz. A couple years ago, I had a skin cancer removed. A melanoma." He pointed to a scar above his left eye. "I even put off going to get that thing checked, and I knew better. Sometimes we doctors are the last ones to take our own advice."

"So you think I have lung cancer. Isn't that pretty unusual? I thought mostly men had lung cancer and more women had breast cancer. After all, I've never smoked."

"Actually, breast cancer might be more common than lung cancer in women, but lung cancer is more lethal. Until a few years ago, breast cancer was considered the most frequent form of cancer among women. But recently I heard that lung cancer probably accounts for the largest number of incidents of cancer. The statistics I heard last week indicate that over 150,000 people are diagnosed with lung cancer each year."

Liz quickly voiced the question that had been hiding in the recesses of her mind. "So tell me the truth, Dr. Franklin. What are the odds of surviving lung cancer?"

The look on Dr. Franklin's face confirmed Liz's suspicions that her chances weren't good. "Lung cancer is really tough, Liz. Statistically, the cure rate is less than one in ten. But let me hasten to add that the rate is improving every year. I personally know at least five people who recently passed their five-year mark and have been declared cured of lung cancer. It isn't easy, but it can be beaten."

Liz sensed a feeling of anger swelling from deep within. *How could this be happening to me? What have I done to deserve this?* A sharp edge was evident in her voice. "I still don't get it, doctor. My dad smoked, but my mom didn't. I don't smoke. My husband doesn't smoke. Even the office where I work is smoke free—there are a few people there who smoke, but they all have to go outside on breaks or use the designated area in the coffee shop in our building."

"That's the thing, Liz," Dr. Franklin replied. "Most cancers are pretty slow to start. In fact, a lot of the research indicates that a cancer may start from a single cell—perhaps it's been affected by tobacco smoke or some other carcinogen—and it starts to change and generate other cells. It may take more than twenty years of cell division to produce a visible tumor. Eventually, if a tumor—that's what we call the mass of cancer cells—goes undetected, or nothing is done to stop its growth, it may eventually take the patient's life. That's why early treatment—using the best medical care available—is so crucial."

Today, with significant treatment strides and heightened public awareness, cancer is becoming less of a killer.

Picking up a writing pad from his desk, Dr. Franklin glanced at his watch, then jotted down a name and address. "I want you to head right over to see Dr. Morris at the oncology clinic. He'll be expecting you. I've asked my nurse to phone and make sure they could get you in today."

A frown creased Liz's face. "You're really taking this seriously, aren't you, Dr. Franklin?"

"It's the only way to take cancer, Liz. I care too much about you to just let it go."

Giving her a kindly pat on the shoulder, he handed her the paper on which he had written the address of the oncology clinic. Then he ushered her out the door. "On your way now, Liz. And remember, your will to fight back will play a big part in how successful your treatment is."

A Sea of Statistics

The grim statistics on cancer show it to be the killer most people consider it to be. But today, with significant treatment strides and heightened public awareness, cancer is becoming less of a killer. Of the four billion people on planet Earth, approximately four million will die from all the different forms of cancer.[3] Twice as many people die from heart attacks and strokes. Approximately one million new cases of cancer are diagnosed each year in the United States, plus more than half a million cases of specialized forms of cancer, such as nonmelanoma skin cancer and highly localized cancers of the cervix and breast in women, cancers that are rarely fatal.

The symptoms Liz experienced—persistent cough and coughing up blood—or other symptoms such as persistent chest pains or audible wheezing, may indicate the presence of lung cancer. The most effective diagnostic technique for lung cancer is a simple chest X ray. If a suspicious mass is noticed, a CAT scan or tomography may provide a more specific diagnosis, as will a biopsy.

Until recent years, the most common form of cancer among women was breast cancer, which affects one out of every nine women. While typically striking women over fifty, breast cancer is also seen in women in their forties or even thirties. There is no single predominant cause indicated for breast cancer, as smoking is with lung cancer. There may be a genetic component, since women whose mothers, sisters, or close female relatives have had the disease seem to be particularly susceptible. Hormonal abnormalities or a diet rich in animal fats may also be factors. Physicians agree that the most effective weapon against breast cancer is early detection. Regular breast self-examination and the mammogram are the key components.

Prostate cancer is extremely common among American men, with more than 100,000 cases diagnosed each year. Gene, who was diagnosed with prostate cancer in his late forties, came from a family where several other members had developed prostate cancer. Researchers at Johns Hopkins University have concluded that men with one or more relatives who have had prostate cancer are up to eleven times more likely to get the disease than men with no family history of the disease. Fortunately for Gene, he had followed his doctor's advice to undergo a rectal exam each year, a procedure recommended by the American Cancer Society for all men over forty.

Prostate cancer often has no symptoms during its earliest stages. Any indications, such as blood in the urine, the need to urinate frequently, or difficulty in starting urination, call for an immediate checkup. Since prostate cancer has a high cure rate, early detection is crucial. The five-year survival rate for prostate cancer has increased to more than 70 percent. However, the need for early detection is underscored by the fact that some 70 percent of prostate tumors spread to other areas of the body before they are detected.

Another common form of cancer many people are frequently reluctant to talk about is cancer of the colon and rectum. The American Cancer Society estimates that more than 90 percent of those diagnosed with this form of cancer could survive past five years with early detection. Former President Ronald Reagan was diagnosed with colon cancer and was successfully treated in 1985. Major risk factors for this kind of cancer include high fat and low fiber diets.

Another major category of cancer includes leukemia and Hodgkin's Disease, a cancer of the lymph nodes. Though these cancers have been among the most deadly in years past, a bone marrow transplant procedure developed a few years ago at M.D. Anderson Hospital in Houston, when coupled with high-dose chemotherapy, has led to a much higher cure rate.

Liz's Emotions

None of these statistics was foremost in Liz's thoughts as she parked her car in the tree-shaded lot next to the oncology clinic. She couldn't help noticing a major hospital on the other side of the parking lot—one of several renowned for treating cancer patients. *I'll probably wind up spending what little time I have left in that hospital,* Liz thought fearfully. *How will I tell my children? What will become of my family?*

Liz had hurriedly phoned her husband, Bill, from Dr. Franklin's office, and, although she had protested, he insisted on meeting her at the oncology clinic. She spotted him standing beside his car in the parking lot when she drove in. Quickly he embraced her, and she found herself fighting back tears.

"It's all right, honey. God will help us lick this thing. You're a fighter." Unable to reply, she simply hugged him hard, while tears brimmed in her eyes. Taking her hand, Bill led Liz into the oncology clinic. A few minutes later they were seated in Dr. Morris's office.

All cancers are actually uncontrolled cell growth.

"You don't look anything like I expected," Liz blurted out uncomfortably. "I sort of thought you'd look like Morris the Cat."

Seated before her was a small, energetic man with a head full of curly black hair, dark sparkling eyes, and a thick mustache. "Not a problem," he said. "In fact, if Morris the Cat were like me, he'd probably be arrested for hyperactivity. That is, assuming you'd arrest a hyperactive cat. He's much more laid back than I am."

Dr. Morris continued almost without pausing. "I know you're both concerned, so I'll get right to the point. Dr. Franklin sent the results of your X rays and scans over. We'll need to do some additional scans in our nuclear medicine department, then do a bronchoscopy so that we can biopsy those cells. There seems to be no doubt that your left lung is pretty involved. I'm hopeful we've caught this early enough so that it hasn't metastasized."

"Metasta . . . does that mean spread?" Liz asked, remembering some of her discussions with her mother's physician.

"Yes. You know, at the risk of being repetitious, maybe the best thing for me to do is to back up to square one—although I suspect Dr. Franklin has already told you a little bit about cancer."

Liz nodded vigorously. "He told me it's more than one disease."

"That's right. In fact, some cancer experts have identified more than a hundred different diseases, or types, of cancer. These all have different characteristics and different treatments. But they do have certain things in common. All cancers are actually uncontrolled cell growth. And cancers can spread through the blood, the lymphatic system—that's sort of the body's drainage system—or even spread by the seeding of body cavities such as the abdomen or a lung. In fact, one of the things we have to be cautious about whenever surgery is performed is to make sure that we don't actually spread the cancer in the process of trying to get rid of it."

Noting the frightened look on his patient's face, Dr. Morris quickly added, "Oh, don't be alarmed. We take extreme care not to spread cancer in this way. The surgeons are trained to utilize what we call 'no touch' techniques. That kind of thing is extremely rare."

As Dr. Morris turned to a chart beside his desk, Liz couldn't help noticing that, like Dr. Franklin's, it too was quite cluttered. She wondered if a cluttered desk was a job hazard for physicians.

"Remember much about your days in high school biology?" Both Liz and Bill shook their heads. "I thought not. Most people don't. But you probably recall that the body is made up of cells, each of which has a fixed number of chromosomes. These cells are constantly splitting. In fact, that's the way our Creator designed us to maintain life and growth."

Bill and Liz quickly glanced at each other. *Could be another Christian doctor*, Liz thought. *I knew Dr. Franklin was a man of faith, but this is almost too much to pray for.*

"There's a lot of variety in cancer cells, or potentially cancerous cells. Some of them look a lot like the original cell types. Some even do some of the same things as normal cells. But they aren't normal. Some are very slow growing and may not cause problems for a long time. Others are referred to as aggressive, or fast growing. They can cause serious health risks if they are not treated immediately.

"Normal cells all have protein markers on their membranes. Each one also has a single nucleus, plus the right number of chromosomes. Cancer cells tend to vary in some way or other from this norm. Now every abnormal cell in a body isn't malignant. For example, you may have scar tissue or warts or even hormone-induced tissue overgrowths. These are forms of what we call neoplastic cells or neoplasms that usually aren't malignant or even harmful." Liz glanced at a wart on the back of her left wrist, while Bill unconsciously touched the scar on his right temple—the product of a childhood fall.

"I see you both can relate. Warts and scar tissue are two good examples of noncancerous neoplasms." As his two guests chuckled nervously, Dr. Morris continued. "I'm sure you've probably heard the terms *benign* and *malignant.* But just to clarify, a benign growth is usually considered harmless. These most commonly are confined in space, grow very slowly, and limit themselves to the area they begin growing in. On the other hand, a malignant growth will usually reproduce more rapidly and has a tendency to invade other parts of the body— that's what we mean by *metastasizing.*

"I remember one man I treated whose cancer started in the colon, then eventually spread to the liver. Nobody thought he would survive—but he did. We usually refer to a cancer by the place where it originates—the technical term, in case you're interested, is *primary lesion.*"

"So my primary lesion would be located in my lung?" Liz asked.

"That's what it looks like."

Raising his hand as if in a classroom at school, Bill asked, "So what are her chances, Doc? What's the prognosis?"

Leaning back in his chair, Dr. Morris stroked his mustache. "To be honest with you, Bill, it's really too early to tell. We need to get the rest of these tests run. Then we'll present Liz's case to a tumor board—that's a panel of cancer specialists who meet on a regular basis to review cancer cases and make recommendations about the best and most up-to-date treatment plans."

"You mean, like a board of directors?" Liz asked, puzzled.

"That's probably as good a way to put it as any." Dr. Morris smiled as he recalled the heated discussion the last time he had sat on a tumor board. "Tumor boards and tumor registries are required by the American College of Surgeons for any hospital cancer treatment program."

Despite her anxiety, Liz couldn't help grinning. "Tumor registries. Tumor boards. Does every cancer patient have to have his or her tumor registered or something?"

"A tumor registry is simply a database of information on the most common forms of cancer. Since a tumor board typically includes surgeons, chemotherapists, pathologists, diagnostic radiologists, and radiotherapists—each of whom has her or her own area of specialty—they need as much information as possible about which forms of cancer are most common in a certain area, which cancers are on the increase, what are the profiles for high-risk and low-risk individuals for different forms of cancer, how different cancers are being treated, and what is the rate of cure. The tumor registry can supply that information. You may be interested to know that there are approximately 800 approved hospital cancer programs with tumor boards and tumor registries around the country."

"So will *you* decide whether or not I have surgery? Or will you ask the board?"

"*I'll* make the final decision, but only after input from the board."

Bill nodded enthusiastically. "I personally like that approach. Not that I don't trust your judgment. It's just that I believe in what Solomon said in Proverbs about the wisdom of a multitude of counselors."

"So you think they'll tell you to operate on me?" Liz tried to swallow the lump in her throat.

---

*Prayer and good medical care
go hand in hand.*

"Back to your question, Bill, about her prognosis. Based on what I've seen in the X rays and scans, I think we're catching this at a pretty good time for Liz. But I suspect we'll have surgery ahead, followed by some pretty intensive treatments. Liz, you probably have already heard from Dr. Franklin that lung cancer is a serious matter."

Squeezing her husband's hand, Liz nodded. She felt close to tears again.

"But I want to be completely candid and realistic with you. Lung cancer is a deadly serious proposition. In fact, any kind of cancer changes the life of the person who has it—changes the lives of their family members too."

Dr. Morris shifted his intent gaze from Liz to Bill. "But I want you both to hear me loud and clear. Cancer is not a death sentence. It's an illness—nothing more, nothing less. I'm convinced that with good medical care, active participation by the patient—and prayer—cancer can be beaten. In fact, nearly half of everyone diagnosed with cancer will be cured. And some cancers, although they can't be cured, are still treatable, so the person can live a relatively normal life."

"Doctor, we're people of faith," Bill said. "We believe in prayer—in miracles. You mentioned prayer. Why can't we just ask God to heal us?"

"You can, and you should. I'm convinced that prayer is essential. From my perspective, it's a key component. My experience is that prayer and good medical care go hand in hand. I've been a Christian ever since I was a teenager. I've directed many patients' care. I always take time to pray and ask God for direction for each one. But in my experience, and that of most other clinicians, it's extremely rare for cancer to disappear without treatment. Medically we'd call that a spontaneous remission. I'm not saying God can't do that. In fact, I've seen many times when a person's recovery went far beyond what we medical people could expect. And I've seen a lot of miracles. But I see them most commonly through a combination of prayer and wise medical care.

"So I hope you're not even thinking of putting off treatment. What I've seen is that, without treatment, cancer continues to grow. Eventually it blocks all the body's important functions, and this leads to death."

Looking intently at Liz, Dr. Morris paused for a moment. "I'm sure you've been wondering if you're going to die of this cancer, Liz." She nodded slowly. "I can't tell you that you won't, but I *can* tell you that we're going to give it our best treatment shot. The additional scans will help confirm that we're making the right diagnosis, as well as pinpoint the tumor's location. When we're absolutely sure of the location, we'll use the bronchoscope to take a biopsy to confirm that it's malignant.

"Then, once we get that confirmation, based on the tumor board's recommendation, we'll go ahead and operate to take out everything we possibly can that's affected by the cancer. The reason we need to move quickly is that you're right at the point where, hopefully, we can contain the malignancy in the one lung. I'm sure you don't have to be told how difficult it would be to survive without at least one lung."

Liz smiled nervously.

"You'll find out a lot more about your treatment as we get into it.* But here's our tentative game plan—just so you'll know. Assuming that the results of the CAT scan and the biopsy are positive, we'll perform surgery to try to remove every possible trace of malignant cells. At this point, that means your left lung. The next step is a series of radiation treatments, or radiotherapy, with which we try to get any malignant cells left by the surgery. Then you might say we mop up with chemotherapy, using some pretty strong chemicals. In fact, our hospital has a wing with a special protective environment where we can carry on intense chemotherapy while minimizing the risk of infection or other side effects."

Dr. Morris rose from his chair, walked to the office window, and pointed to the sun setting in the west, juxtaposed against a bank of storm clouds. Then he turning to Liz and her husband. "I guess there's a sense in which your prognosis looks a lot like the weather out there. There's some dark clouds —the type of cancer you have is quite serious—but there are some bright spots as well. I don't think your cancer is so far advanced that it's spread from the left lung. Generally, you seem to be physically fit. I didn't notice any other medical conditions or complications like diabetes on your chart.

"Quite frankly, one of the big factors in surviving cancer is your will to live. We doctors can give you sort of an educated guess as to how well you will do, based on statistics. But the three most important factors to keep in mind are the will to live on your part, getting good medical care, and your faith in God."

The room was quiet for a moment, then Bill spoke up. "So how do we cope with this monster that's invaded our lives? Liz and I are pretty strong people, but, man, this is a lot!"

* We will discuss more specific treatments in chapter 8.

Dr. Morris nodded his head sympathetically. "I know, Bill. I really don't enjoy sharing this kind of news with anyone—even though I've had to do it hundreds of times. It's never fun telling someone they're going to have to cope with cancer. So let me share a few basic tips that will help you.

"First, educate yourself. There are a lot of good books out there on the subject, a lot of clinical books, question-and-answer type books. Before today, neither of you would probably have been very interested in them. But now I'd encourage you to read, to ask questions, to find out everything you can about treatment options. That way you can really take charge of your own recovery—sort of appoint yourself the captain of your recovery team. But be realistic about your options, and be careful of some of the things people will suggest to you. Also, it's important to remember that sometimes test results can give you several distinctively different options. So don't hesitate to ask me and the other doctors questions. In fact, I'll be encouraging you to ask. Some patients even tape my answers; others take notes.

"The second area that's important to face is your emotions. You'll find that a lot of people around you won't understand your feelings. In fact, this will be true for both of you. But feel free to express your feelings, even when people don't understand."

Dr. Morris walked around to the front of his desk. "Cry when you feel like crying, Liz. Tears are a natural part of the recovery process. Oh, and another thing, I recommend that you put together a list of relatives and friends you can look to as a sort of support network. You may even want to draw up a list of their names and telephone numbers. After all, you can't be sure when you may need someone—maybe even just to talk to. You'll be hearing more about support groups—the hospital has a list of groups that meet throughout this area. I'd encourage you to consider joining one."

Bill and Liz sat numbly as Dr. Morris continued. "Another thing I like to tell patients early in the process is to be careful not to confuse the negative side effects of treatment with the illness itself. Some of the medication you may take, the chemotherapy, may produce pretty bad side effects at times. It's important to make sure that you keep those separate in your thinking from the cancer itself so that you don't become too discouraged."

Noticing that Liz seemed to be staring at her hands, which were held rigidly in her lap, Dr. Morris paused. Noticing the silence, she looked up, tears rimming her eyes. "What's the point?" she asked intensely. "Maybe my purpose in life is over. Maybe this is God's way of telling me it's time to die."

"I think I understand how you feel. I've talked to a lot of people who react just about like you when they first get the news that cancer has become a part of their lives. Let me suggest a simple test to find out if your purpose in life has been completed. Take a deep breath." The doctor paused as Liz followed his instructions. "Now let it out and take another."

Puzzled, Liz shook her head. "I don't get it. What does this have to do with my purpose in life?"

Dr. Morris smiled. "It's really simple, Liz. If you can still breathe, you have life. And that means your purpose in life isn't completed yet. Oh, and one other thing—see that plaque on the wall? That's the key to the whole process."

Walking to the wall, he removed the plaque and placed it in Liz's hand. She looked down at it and quietly read the words:

> God grant me the Serenity
> to accept the things I cannot change,
> the Courage to change the things I can,
> and the Wisdom to know the difference.

She stared intently at the plaque before her for a moment, then glanced at her husband before turning to Dr. Morris. "The serenity prayer, eh? I sure don't feel very serene right now."

"I'm sure you don't. I didn't feel very serene when I first found out I had cancer either."

Both Bill and Liz sat upright as though jolted by an electric wire. Liz was the first to speak. "You . . . had . . . cancer? But you're an oncologist. A cancer doctor."

"Oncologists are susceptible to cancer too. Seven years ago I discovered that I had prostate cancer. Things didn't sound very promising. I found out firsthand what I had only known from medical classes and textbooks. But last summer I passed my five-year cure mark. And I think my cancer played a key role in two very important events in my life.

"First, it was through my cancer that I met the man who ultimately led me to the most important relationship in my life—my faith in Jesus Christ. And it was during this time that I began to grow in my faith. That's when I learned the true meaning of the serenity prayer. I had heard it before—I was a recovering alcoholic. I became involved in a twelve-step group when I was in medical school. So I had prayed the prayer often.

"But it was only when I came to understand what Christ had done for me—what His death and resurrection meant to me personally—that I learned how to trust Him, to accept the things I couldn't change, and to let Him strengthen me to change the things I could."

"And for the wisdom to know the difference?" Liz asked.

"Exactly," Dr. Morris replied.

3

A PERSPECTIVE ON PHYSICAL ILLNESS

D on, it's every parent's nightmare." There was a catch in the voice of the tall, blue-eyed man with sandy hair who sat in the booth of a well-known Dallas barbecue restaurant. He was relating a story that would touch the heartstrings of any parent. "Every parent dreads some major catastrophe happening to his child. Every parent fears losing a child."

Ron and his wife, Dianna, had lived with this nightmare for the past two years. Their twelve-year-old daughter, Jessica, had been given absolutely no hope of recovering from osteogenic sarcoma—a fairly rare type of bone cancer. Their experiences raised the question as old as the patriarch Job: Why?

Why an innocent young girl? Why a virtual death sentence? Why? Why? Why?

Through our experiences with the practice of medicine, psychiatry, and oncology nursing, as well as teaching, pastoral ministry, and counseling, we have faced this question hundreds—perhaps thousands—of times.

Why physical illness? Why tragedy? More to the point, why me? Why my daughter? Why my child? Why my loved one?

No Simple Answers

Philosophers and theologians have grappled with these issues for centuries, yet no one has come up with an easy, simple answer. There simply is no sugarcoating for that most difficult of pills for the human race to swallow—unexplained and unexplainable adversity, sickness, suffering, even death.

That was the question with which Ron and his wife, Dianna, had been forced to deal, but not in terms of abstract philosophical concepts or pious platitudes to be shared with others as a part of vocational ministry. For even though Ron had spent years as a pastor, he and his wife were now forced to wrestle with the kind of pain and adversity many people only experience in their worst nightmares.

But this was no nightmare. It was real.

Jessica's tragic illness came crashing down on the Eggert family just after Ron had been put in a position of ministering to one of his best friends, whose eighteen-year-old son had been murdered. "At the funeral service, I really sought to point the family to God, to encourage confidence in Him. That was the theme of my message. And at the time, everybody of course was asking 'Why?' Why this? What happened? Why would God allow this?"

Running his fingers through his thinning hair, Ron smiled. "Little did I know then. It's almost ironic. The theme of my message was *You Don't Need to Know Why If You Know Who.* If you know God intimately enough and if you understand who He is—if you accept His sovereignty as well as His love and His grace—you really don't need to wrestle with why. You just trust Him. But trusting Him is one thing when it's someone else's child who has died an untimely death. It's another when you have just heard a death sentence pronounced for your youngest child."

Jessica

It was the summer of 1990. Ron and Dianna, exhausted from the demands of ministry, had taken their four children on a much needed vacation. "I remember it like it was yesterday," Ron said. "We had stopped for lunch at a coffee shop. While we were waiting to be seated, Dianna reached over to hug Jessica. She felt a lump just above her collarbone."

The next morning Ron and Dianna took Jessica to a clinic in Salem, Oregon, where the lump was X-rayed. Within two hours, Ron and Dianna's worst fears were realized.

"The doctor took us aside into a little room. His secretary took Jessica out to ask her how she spelled her name. That was a dead giveaway. The doctor didn't waste any time beating around the bush. He said, 'This one is nasty. You've got to get home immediately.' We asked, 'Well, can't you just figure out what it is here?'" Ron paused, glanced out a nearby window, and stroked his chin. "That doctor didn't want to fool with it. He told us, 'You need the continuity of care. This is nasty. It's serious. It's an emergency. Get home immediately!' So we did."

A rushed trip home was followed by two days of intensive tests. Then came another conference, this one with the Eggert's new oncologist, John Champion. "Our doctor has been open and up front with us the whole time. No beating around the bush. No surprises later. He met with us in his office and simply said, 'Here's *what* it is. Here's *where* it is. Here's what it looks like on the X rays. Here are the patterns of what we would expect to see. And it's already way down the line.'"

What Ron and Dianna learned was that osteogenic sarcoma starts in a limb—a leg or an arm. The cancer cells cause the growth in bones to go wild. The normal response is to immediately amputate the limb before the cancer has a chance to spread to the chest and lungs, then follow up with a series of aggressive chemotherapy treatments.

"By the time we discovered Jessica's cancer, it was behind her heart. It was in her lungs. There were already a half-dozen tumors—including three or four tumors in her chest. It was too late to amputate."

Ron paused, then continued as a tightness crept into his voice. "The doctor showed us X rays of how the tumor had surrounded her trachea and esophagus, and all those blood vessels. He didn't mince words. He said, 'You know, that's going to choke off her air supply quickly. It will take her life. We're going to take an extremely aggressive treatment of chemotherapy. That's all we can do. These are the four drugs we will use, and these are the side effects.'"

The doctor answered the unspoken question that hung ominously in their minds. "You need to sign these papers because you have *got* to do this. If not, your daughter has two months to live. If we do this aggressive chemotherapy, all we can hope for is to buy six or eight months. But that's presupposing that we totally stop the growth of the major tumor. Quite frankly, these don't usually stop growing. We may be able to slow it down with chemotherapy, but there's no cure for this. And there's rarely any remission for this kind of cancer. We'll buy her a little time. We'll try to relieve her pain. In fact, she's likely to be in excruciating pain. But I can't promise any quality of life."

Hardly believing what they were hearing, Ron and Dianna listened as the doctor concluded the interview. "We'll do our best to buy her some time and do the best we can to make her comfortable. That's all we can do."

As Ron reflected back on the personal trauma of hearing that his youngest daughter had virtually no chance of surviving this disease, he put it into statistical perspective. "The interesting thing was, people in the hospital would come up to us, upset and crying because their doctor only gave their child an 80 percent chance to live, or maybe 50 percent. Our doctor never gave Jessica any hope of living. He said he might give her a 4 percent chance of lasting a year, a 1 percent chance of making it two years. That was the same as saying there was no chance. We had to address it. We had to deal with it. We were forced to accept the inevitability of her death."

Sickness and death. A child dying of cancer. A successful major league baseball pitcher losing an arm because of a malignant tumor. A famous singer-songwriter, a noted actor, a talented musician. The names are familiar to us: Dave Dravecky, Roger Miller, Michael Landon, Dizzy Gillespie.

Then there are the names of people we know—parents, cousins, uncles and aunts, spouses, business colleagues, close friends . . . even children. And we continue to ask, "Why?"

Sickness and Scripture

Though the subject of cancer isn't specifically addressed in Scripture, the theme of sickness permeates both the Old and New Testaments. Job suffered from incredibly painful boils.

Moses' sister, Miriam, contracted leprosy. The infant son born to David and Bathsheba became critically ill, then died. Naaman the Syrian sought a cure for his leprosy in Israel. Nebuchadnezzar, king of Babylon, developed a mental disorder that resulted in bizarre behavior. King Hezekiah became seriously ill.

It has been observed that almost 20 percent of the four gospel accounts of the life of Christ address the topic of sickness and healing.[1] Whereas this is not the major focus of the New Testament message (the death and resurrection of Christ is), the subject receives significant attention there and throughout the history of the early church as recorded in the book of Acts (8:7; 19:11–12; 28:3–10). Paul addresses his own illness in 2 Corinthians 12:7–10. A procedure for dealing with physical illness and its effects is outlined in James 5:13–16.

Scripture makes clear that every
incidence of illness is not a direct
result of some specific sin
or of a spiritual deficiency.

The subject of physical illness has also played a prominent role in secular history. Historical records indicate that bone cancer was identified in mummies in the great pyramid of Gaza between 2500 and 1500 B.C.[2] The famous Greek physician Hippocrates, whose name is linked to the oath that used to be taken by every physician, coined the term *carcinoma* to refer to spreading tumors that can take a patient's life. Hippocrates and, two centuries later, Galen (a physician who practiced and taught medicine in Rome) both subscribed to what is commonly called the *humoral theory* of disease, which based medical treatment on the condition of humors, or bodily fluids. They considered blood from the heart, phlegm from the head, yellow bile from the liver, and black bile from the spleen to be the key components of health. According to this theory, diseases resulted from an imbalance of these four humors. Interestingly, Galen held the opinion that melancholy women were more susceptible to breast cancer than sanguine women, a view supported by psychological research today.[3]

From a biblical perspective, several key observations can be made. First, sickness is a major factor in human existence because of man's fall into sin. When Adam and Eve defied God's instruction and decided to take the forbidden fruit, they triggered God's dire prediction that "in the day that you eat of it, you shall surely die" (Genesis 2:17).

Though that prediction was not fulfilled immediately (it would be in due time), physical sickness, and ultimately death, have been the common experience of humans ever since our first parents. Nowhere is this more evident than in the fifth chapter of Genesis, a section labeled "The Book of the Generations of Adam." Eight times in thirty-two verses the pronouncement is made, "and he died." Like a phonograph needle stuck in the groove of a defective record, the passage reverberates with this gloomy note—a fact observed by Paul in his comment that "death reigned from Adam to Moses" (Romans 5:14).

Although the Bible is not a medical textbook, it does refer directly or indirectly to a wide range of illnesses with both physical and emotional components, including blindness, deafness, epilepsy, fever, hemorrhaging, indigestion, weakness, leprosy, palsy, and many more.[4] However, Scripture makes clear that every incidence of illness is not a direct result of some specific sin or of a spiritual deficiency such as a lack of faith.

Some time ago a young pastor went to visit a member of his parish the night before she was scheduled for major surgery. Seating himself beside her bed in what he supposed to be a comforting posture, he began his conversation with the words, "Now let's see if we can figure out what sin in your life has brought on this illness."

Sadly, this young minister's misconception of the relationship between specific illness and sin is shared by many individuals today. And it was also held by no less a group than the disciples of Jesus. One of those men, John, candidly describes an incident in the ninth chapter of his gospel. It was a tense moment in the life of Christ—He had just confronted the religious leaders of His day with His divinity, asserting that "before Abraham was, I am" (John 8:58). That His protagonists understood the message is evident from their response—they took up stones to cast at Him. Remarkably, Jesus was able to become lost in the crowd, getting away without harm.

Yet even in this tense moment, Christ didn't fail to notice an individual sitting in the temple courtyard, a man who had been blind since birth. The disciples noticed also and asked Jesus a question commonly echoed even by some godly individuals today: "Rabbi, who sinned, this man or his parents, that he was born blind?" (John 9:2). Jesus' immediate response laid to rest any notion that every instance of illness can be traced to some specific spiritual weakness or sin: "Neither this man nor his parents sinned, but that the works of God should be revealed in him" (v. 3).

Why Sickness and Suffering?

Over lunch one afternoon, a minister and a psychiatrist who were close friends began discussing instances of illness with which they were familiar—family members and close friends. As the discussion progressed, they began listing on paper napkins every reason they could think of for illness and physical suffering.

Perhaps the most important reason for suffering could be described as "reason known to God but not given to man."

By the time the list they developed was published,[5] the number of causes had grown to seventeen. Some instances were clearly a consequence of sin, such as the death of David's young baby. Still others were part of God's loving discipline of His children (Hebrews 12:5–11).

However, many physical adversities are simply designed to strengthen our faith, while producing steadfastness, approved character, and hope (Romans 5:3–4); others are meant to give us a means of encouraging people in their adversity (2 Corinthians 1:3–4); some give evidence or "show the proof" of our faith (1 Peter 1:3–9); sometimes suffering develops such positive character qualities as humility (2 Corinthians 12:7) or simply glorifies God, as in the case of the man who was born blind (John 9:3).

Perhaps the most important reason for suffering could be described as "reason known to God but not given to man."[6] That was the case in the life of the patriarch Job. After suffering a series of incredible disasters that left his financial empire in ruins and all his children dead in the aftermath of a tragic storm, Job developed a serious illness—incredibly painful boils. The combination of itching and intense pain left him absolutely miserable. Furthermore, he was isolated from social contact, since his body was covered with open sores.

Why had this happened? Totally unknown to Job, God in His sovereignty had permitted Satan to attack the patriarch's family and personal health. Satan was sure that if he were allowed to carry out this attack, Job would renounce God. Job's wife actually encouraged her husband to do this very thing! Yet God in His omniscience was equally sure that, despite the difficulty of the test, Job would ultimately "come forth as gold" (Job 23:10). Obviously God was correct.

Scripture makes clear that those who teach that individuals who become sick are always in sin or out of the will of God or deficient in faith are wrong. However, this observation immediately raises other important questions: How can a good God allow suffering? How can an all-powerful God not take action to stop the suffering of those He loves? These are the questions addressed by Christian writer and philosopher C. S. Lewis, who lost the love of his life—his wife, Joy Gresham—to cancer shortly after they were married.

Two years after her death from cancer of the leg and breast, Lewis penned a classic volume titled *The Problem of Pain,* in which he addressed those towering questions. If God is good, why does He permit suffering? If He is all-powerful, why doesn't He prevent it?

Lewis had lived with the same nightmare faced by Ron and Dianna. He had cried out to his beloved in her pain and sickness, "Don't leave me, Joy!" Following her death, Lewis honestly struggled with feelings of hurt, anger, and pain. "I turned to God, now that I really needed Him. And what do I find? A door slammed in my face. The sound of bolting. And after that . . . silence."[7]

Cliff and his family were forced to grapple with the "why" question when he was diagnosed with colon cancer. A tall, thin college professor, Cliff was known as a people person, despite his natural shyness. He enjoyed interacting with his students— even becoming involved in an occasional pickup game of basketball.

When told he had cancer of the colon, Cliff utilized his strong faith and sense of humor to cope with the ordeal before him. As he put it the evening before he was to undergo surgery, "I'll come out of this with a semi-colon."

For a time it seemed that the combination of surgery, radiotherapy, and chemotherapy had defeated the cancer. Then things took a turn for the worse. The diagnosis: liver metastasis. The prognosis: not good. At this point, Cliff's doctors were measuring his life expectancy in months.

Yet five years later, Cliff is still alive. A recent checkup declared his cancer to be in remission. Although by his own admission not in the best of health, he nonetheless considers that things could be much worse.

Sitting in the living room of his comfortable suburban home, Cliff took a deep sip from a glass of iced tea. "Sure I wondered why. I imagine we all do in these kinds of circumstances. But I didn't dwell on the question because I knew there was no answer. After all, if you're going to ask 'Why me?' when trouble comes, you have to ask 'Why me?' when good things happen. None of us really deserves anything. Whatever we have comes our way by the grace of God. That's certainly true of salvation, but it's true of physical health as well.

"I have a brother who's never been sick a day in his life. I don't have a clue as to why all this has happened to me and he's been spared. All I know is, I can trust God. Not only does He have a reason for the sickness, He provides grace for the pain and the suffering as well. God has been good to give me strength through these years. He's also been good to give me faith to trust Him for healing. Even though there's the threat of recurrence, I'm still convinced that, to a great degree, it's safe to say I've been healed of my cancer."

Healing by Faith

It's impossible to talk about sickness and adversity without addressing the subject of healing by faith. In the opinion of the authors, two extremes are frequently taken regarding faith and healing. One is to insist on an instant miracle, an immediate cure. Some would even go so far as to say that efforts to seek medical care should be dropped in favor of faith and healing. At the other end of the spectrum are those who simply see prayer and faith as placebos for pain and sickness. Their rationalistic presuppositions dictate that in our modern world medical care is the only real answer.

Our personal experience and conviction is that neither extreme is appropriate. Rather, what we need is a balance composed of three ingredients:

- an absolute trusting confidence in God's ability to heal
- a willingness to vigorously pursue the best available medical care
- the conviction that, whatever happens, God is both good and sovereign—too good to allow anything ultimately to happen to us that is not in our best interest and too powerful to be frustrated in His purposes for our lives

BACK TO JESSICA

Jessica not only underwent chemotherapy but eventually multiple surgeries as well. Ron and Dianna were quick to acknowledge the miracles during the two-year course of young Jessica's illness. They were equally quick to recognize the role played by the best available medical care. As Ron sat in the booth in the barbecue stand in Dallas chronicling the story of his family's ordeal, he shared two anecdotes that illustrated this balance. Both related to physicians involved in Jessica's care.

"The oncologist who first told us Jessica's case was hopeless—that there was no way she would survive—was young, maybe in his early forties. He had two children of his own. He was a neat dresser, very personable—sort of a hang-loose kind of doctor. We've been extremely pleased with his care.

"He was part of a strange thing that happened after Jessica's arm surgery. One of the secretaries, or a nurse, was really into all this nutrition stuff about cancer. She kept telling us we needed to get Jessica on vitamins, vegetable juice, that kind of thing. Kept insisting that she get us some material from the research she had done.

"Dianna told her, 'You know, Jessica's diet isn't all that bad. When she gets out of the hospital, she wants a steak and baked potato and a big tossed salad. She's always liked healthy food. Her favorite food is a big, fresh vegetable plate—carrots, celery, cauliflower, broccoli.'

"So the nurse says, 'Boy, that's probably why Jessica is doing so well. Must be nutrition or that diet she's been eating.' So later Dianna asked the doctor, 'Hey, what do you think about nutrition? How big a part do you think that's played in Jessica's recovery? She does have a good, nutritional diet, you know.'

"I've no doubt that prayer has been the key to Jessica's survival," Ron stated without hesitation.

"The doctor just kind of smiled and said, 'Well, it can't hurt anything. But seriously, Dianna, that couldn't begin to explain Jessica's situation. There's been another force at work in her case. I've had patients with good diets who didn't recover anywhere near like what Jessica's doing.'"

Zero chance of long-term recovery—that's what this same specialist had told Jessica's parents. Four or five tumors in Jessica's chest. One surrounding her trachea, another her esophagus. The largest tumor, the one behind her heart, they considered totally inoperable. Less than a 4 percent chance of surviving a year, 1 percent to live two years.

Now, more than two years later, Jessica has celebrated her thirteenth birthday. Her long, straight, blonde hair, which had fallen out during her treatments, came back brown and curly. She still had to undergo multiple surgeries, plus intensive chemotherapy treatments.

But she is alive!

"I've no doubt that prayer has been the key to Jessica's survival," Ron stated without hesitation. "During the three major surgeries we faced over the last several months, our church set up a twenty-four-hour prayer vigil each time. A lady in the church made up a chart so people could sign up for fifteen-minute segments. They did this around the clock for three days during the surgeries. Talk about encouraging! Some people

signed up for a whole hour. Families would take an hour—
sometimes each of the children would have a fifteen minute
time slot.

"Then there were people who phoned, literally from all
over the country! A couple of staff members of Focus on the
Family phoned us regularly. People from other ministries.
Friends from all over. That certainly encouraged our faith."

JESUS THE HEALER

So how does faith operate in cases of physical illness?
When we examine the New Testament, we discover that faith
plays a key role. That's what happened to the woman who for
twelve years had a chronic, seemingly incurable, hemorrhage.
Having spent all her resources on medical care, she actually
grew worse.

Finally, in desperation mixed with trust, she came up to
Jesus in the security of a crowd: "If only I may touch His
clothes, I shall be made well" (Mark 5:27–28). When she
touched His clothing, two things immediately occurred: first,
her incurable hemorrhage immediately dried up—she knew in
her body that she had been healed; second, Jesus, knowing
that someone had tapped His power, turned about and said,
"Who touched My clothes?" (vv. 29–30).

His disciples were astounded. "You see the multitude
thronging You, and You say, 'Who touched Me?'" (v. 31).

Yet Mark records that "He looked around to see her who
had done this thing." When she explained what had happened,
He told her, "Daughter"—the only time in the New Testament
Jesus responded to a woman with this term—"your faith has
made you well" (vv. 32–34).

Sometimes, as in this case, it is the faith of the individual
who is sick that makes him well. At other times it may be the
faith of someone else. At the point in His life when He was
interrupted by the woman with the issue of blood, Jesus was en
route to the home of a synagogue official named Jairus, whose
daughter was at the point of death (vv. 22–23). When told by
some of His associates not to bother coming since Jairus's
daughter was dead, Jesus responded with words of encouragement. "Do not be afraid; only believe" (v. 36). Ultimately, Jairus's
faith was rewarded. Jesus restored his daughter to life.

In a similar incident earlier in Jesus' ministry, Mark records the story of a paralytic brought by four friends while He was speaking in a home in Capernaum. Their faith—persistent to the point of digging a hole in the flat roof to let the paralytic down into Jesus' presence—was rewarded. Mark clearly notes, "When Jesus saw *their* faith," He restored the man to health.

On other occasions Jesus healed when *no one* evidenced faith. At His arrest in the garden of Gethsemane, Peter pulled out a sword and sliced the ear from the head of the servant of the high priest. Luke, a physician, identified it as the man's right ear (Luke 22:50). In response to no one's faith, Jesus simply said, "Permit me," touched the servant's ear, and instantly healed the man of his injury.

Thus, the biblical record shows healing in response to faith—the faith of a sick individual or the faith of those close to a sick person—and even healing in response to no one's faith.

NOT HEALED

Ironically, Scripture also presents one example of an individual of great faith—a man who was able to heal others—yet who was never healed himself. We are not told the specific nature of Paul's malady—he refers to it as "a thorn in the flesh" and a "messenger of Satan" (2 Corinthians 12:7). Yet this apostle, who according to Acts 19:11–12 was able to cure the illnesses of others even from a distance, asked God three times for healing. And three times God said no (2 Corinthians 12:8–9).

So what happened here? Surely Paul was a man of great faith. Yet it clearly was not God's purpose to cure him, to heal him. Without question, those who insist that it's always God's will to heal and that we must be guilty of some sin or lack of faith whenever we are not healed haven't considered the implications of Paul's personal experience as recorded in 2 Corinthians.

In acknowledging his lack of healing, Paul gives a clear indication of God's purpose behind his illness. In doing so, the apostle identifies three of the reasons the pastor and the psychiatrist included in their list of why Christians sometimes suffer and become ill.

First, Paul notes that God allowed this illness to keep him from becoming proud. Paul had just finished telling about an incredible experience God had permitted him. Speaking in the third person he told of being caught up into the very presence of God, hearing and seeing things humans will never experience this side of glory. Aware that even such a godly apostle could become "exalted above measure" (v. 7), God lovingly permitted this physical adversity to keep the apostle humble.

It isn't possible for us to always distinguish between what God permits and what Satan causes.

How gracious of our God to provide tangible reminders that all we have and are is of Him, that it isn't our ability or prowess that is ultimately responsible for any success. Lee Iacocca generally has been recognized as one of the most successful CEOs in American industry. Almost single-handedly, he turned Chrysler around from a company that required hundreds of millions of dollars in federal bail-out money to a profitable automotive entity, competitive with the other domestic and import manufacturers. By his own admission, Iacocca's success at Chrysler grew directly out of an incredibly painful experience—his firing as president of Ford Motor Company. Sometimes a disaster or illness can keep us humble, while preparing us for future growth and success.

The second factor Paul observed behind his suffering was spiritual conflict. The apostle considered his ailment to be a "messenger of Satan," perhaps trying to urge him to give up. Without question, Satan's agenda is to do everything he can to remove the effectiveness of our faith. That was his agenda with Job, certainly with Paul, and probably with young Jessica and her family as well.

It isn't possible for us to always distinguish between what God permits and what Satan causes. And though we are frequently tempted to say, "God, why have you allowed the hedge to be moved in so uncomfortably close, so painfully near?" we can rest assured of the incredible contrast between the character and integrity of God and the vicious, self-serving objectives of the accuser of the brethren, characterized by Peter as a hungry lion looking for people to devour (1 Peter 5:8). Continued awareness of Satan's vicious motive can prompt us to follow Peter's exhortation to remain steadfast in faith, utilizing the resources of prayer (v. 7) and the encouragement of others, much as Jessica's family did.

Jessica, Dave, and Melissa

"There were so many who encouraged us," Ron reminisced as he sipped his iced tea. "Dave Dravecky even called following one of the surgeries, just to talk with Jessica. She was asleep after receiving chemotherapy, but Dave spent half an hour talking with Dianna. He was such an encouragement. Then later, when he was in Dallas on a tour to promote his book, he took time to visit with Jessica.

"Then someone put us in touch with Melissa Gilbert of *Little House on the Prairie* fame. Jessica was making copies one day at a nearby office. One of the men who worked there asked about her. When he discovered that one of her favorite television shows was *Little House,* he began making contacts with people he knew in Los Angeles. Then an airline donated tickets, and Melissa Gilbert herself arranged to have a limousine meet us at the airport. We spent four days at her home and met several members of the cast of *Little House*—all of whom had been affected by the death of Michael Landon from pancreatic cancer the previous summer.

"Melissa Gilbert and her husband—all the people we met there were so friendly, so down-to-earth. I'm convinced their interest in Jessica was genuine—it wasn't some publicity stunt. And those are just a couple of the thousands of acts of encouragement and kindness. People coming to the hospital, preparing food, contributing to help defray expenses."

Most important of all, as Jessica's father affirmed while recounting his family's two-year ordeal, God had a purpose. He somehow intended to use this terrible tragedy to glorify Himself.

When asked how he and his wife had dealt with the numbing shock of first hearing the news, Ron responded, "Honestly, we prayed two things. We sat down together and said, hey, we know God can do a miracle. But apart from a miracle, we're going to lose Jessica. We know that God can answer prayer. But we also know that Christians die—good Christians. Even Christians who really know how to pray. So we said to the Lord, 'Lord, we don't understand what You're doing. We don't know what's ahead. We don't know what You plan to do. And we sure don't understand why. But that's not critical, because we trust You.

"'But Lord, we want to ask You two things. First, it would be our prayer, our great desire, that Jessica not have to suffer unduly. If you're going to take her home, take her home. But we would certainly ask that she would not have to suffer unduly.' Second, we prayed, 'God whatever You have in mind, whatever You're going to do, You receive glory through Jessica's situation.'" According to Ron Eggert, God answered both those requests in clear-cut fashion.

Incredible Answers to Prayer for Jessica

From the very beginning, Jessica's oncologist was amazed at how little pain she experienced. Ron remembered his words: "We know her life will be short. We can't even promise any quality of life. Usually, by the time cancer is as involved as Jessica's, the pain is unbearable." But for some reason, Jessica wasn't experiencing any significant pain.

"Then she had this arm surgery," Ron continued. "It was supposed to take eight hours. It lasted more than twelve. The doctor took out two-thirds of her humerus bone—the bone that connects her shoulder with her elbow—and replaced it. And they took out half of her shoulder. Afterwards they gave her this morphine push thing so that she could overcome the incredible pain they anticipated. But she never even needed it! She took one Tylenol the day after the operation. Never a twinge of pain from the cancer. None of the excruciating pain the doctors said she would have. You talk about God answering prayer!"

And what about God receiving glory from this tragic circumstance? Ron ticked off on his fingers his observation of how God had received glory. "First, God has spared her life for over two years, and her story has literally gone around the world. The local newspapers have interviewed us. She's been talked about on both secular and Christian media. What God has done to miraculously save her life has been a remarkable testimony to His power.

"Second, her spirit has been an incredible testimony—and a real encouragement to all of us around her. I think her cheerful spirit in the face of this whole ordeal has really glorified Him.

"Third, I think God has also been glorified through our family's response. The other three children and Dianna have responded so well." Ron described how he and Dianna had been "just real up-front" with the other three kids. "We sought to communicate our confidence in God to them. They've grown spiritually through it."

Adding up a total of thirty-six hospital stays over a two-year period, Ron observed how his other children have grown not only spiritually but in personal maturity as well. "They've all been incredible. Everybody has pitched in. They all know how to iron—the boys iron their own shirts. With their mother staying at the hospital with Jessica for weeks, she couldn't possibly keep up with everything."

Pausing for another sip of his iced tea, Ron shifted position, a smile stretching across his still-youthful face. "Then there were the seemingly little incidents during the ordeal in which the sovereign, loving hand of God was clearly evident. First, there was the matter of our insurance. Two and a half years ago, I had become sick and tired of my insurance. I wasn't happy with the coverage. My insurance group was changing carriers on me every six months—or so it seemed. I was pastoring at the time. I talked to my elders about it."

*"He was the ideal doctor
to perform this particular operation."*

Ron suggested they set him up with a savings account of about $10,000, permit him to drop his health insurance, and self-insure. They said, "Hey, Eggert, you've got four kids. You can't do that. That would be dumb."

"And I said, 'OK, you're probably right.' So they suggested I apply to Kaiser, see if I could get into their HMO. They told me I probably wouldn't get it because all they do is group stuff but to go ahead and apply anyway.

"Well, I did, and I was accepted the first of July. Jessica was diagnosed on July 24, and Kaiser has covered virtually 100 percent of our medical costs. We pay ten dollars per doctor visit, and for the first three blood transfusions in a year—and that's all.

"I haven't the foggiest notion of what our total medical expenses have been. I'm convinced it's close to half a million dollars. Every hospitalization runs between ten and twelve thousand dollars, the surgeries much more. We've also seen God's hand even in meeting our other major expenses—our phone bills, meals in the cafeteria, gasoline for trips to the hospital. The Lord has provided just what we needed—and often just at the point when it's been due."

Ron detailed yet another evidence of God's gracious control over the situation. "When Jessica talked to Dave Dravecky, we all expected she was going to have her arm amputated—in fact, we went into the surgery actually believing she would lose her arm. Then at the last minute the insurance company refused to authorize the surgeon who was to do the amputation. So we had to get another surgeon, and we thought, *Oh, great!*"

So Ron and Dianna met with a different surgeon, Dr. Andrei A. Czitrom, a clinical associate professor in the department of orthopedic surgery at the University of Texas Southwestern Medical Center. "He's one of the very few surgeons in the world who does this procedure—travels all over the world teaching, conducting seminars about it. Turned out he was the ideal doctor to perform this particular operation."

Ron went on to explain why. "Instead of Jessica losing her arm as we had expected, he was able to save the arm, utilizing a bone transplant technique he had developed to connect her shoulder bone to the elbow with a prosthesis and new bone. It turned out she lost some tissue in her shoulder and some mobility in the upper arm, but she still has the use of her hand and her forearm."

A big smile spread across Ron's face as he reminisced about what had been a very traumatic time. "We went to see this Dr. Czitrom. We were pretty discouraged, because he started off talking to us about how amputation is a very radical procedure, has a traumatic effect on the whole body, and it's never the same. We're thinking he's saying, 'Hey, I'm sorry. We just can't do anything.' So we interrupt him and say, 'Wait a minute. Do we have a choice? We don't want to just give up. The other doctor said if we don't take the arm off, it's going to keep spreading until it kills her!'

"Dr. Czitrom said, 'No, no. You misunderstand. I'm talking about saving the arm. I'm going to do the surgery, but I believe I can save the arm.' So he spends the next three hours with us. Pulls a medical textbook off the shelf, shows us the picture of the procedure he's going to do. How he plans to take two-thirds of the humerus bone, then replace it with a bone from a bone bank and a prosthesis, like a big tent stake, going all the way through the bone. When he shut the medical textbook, I noticed his name on the front. He wrote the text! I mean, you just can't beat it!" By this time Ron's grin had turned into a genuine, heartfelt laugh.

"Later Dr. Czitrom recommended another surgeon, Dr. Michael Mack, who's pioneered a technique of video assisted surgeries to go into the chest cavity using just a little four-inch incision with another half-inch incision above it through which he put a plastic tube with a camera lens at the end of it."

Another smile crosses Ron's face. "We went home and told Jessica, and the rest of our family decided to call it Nintendo surgery. This guy is the head of a thirteen-doctor surgical team here in the Dallas/Fort Worth Metroplex. He's the doctor who pioneered using this technique in the chest. I guess you could say he's on the cutting edge of surgical techniques." Again Ron laughed. Then he turned serious.

"I guess to sum it all up, it's been incredibly difficult. There have been times we've been pretty discouraged, even to the point of utter exhaustion. It's been like a roller coaster, so many ups and downs. But now, we're talking about Jessica being tumor free. They don't use the term *cancer free* because they don't know where there may be microscopic cancer cells that have spread. That's why we're still doing chemotherapy.

"But we never expected in a hundred years that we would get to the point of having so many of these tumors out and for her to be so close to being tumor free. We don't know what the future holds. This kind of cancer could crop up at any time. And we still don't understand why. But somehow the Lord has brought us through it all, one day at a time. We've learned to live what I had shared with others. We don't know why, but we do know Who."

4

How Do You Get Cancer?

L ife, with all its surprises, can seem almost insignificant to the child who has everything. And Angela had just about everything a child could want—a loving family, a nice home, times of fun, and plenty of friends with whom to share them. Reflecting back on her childhood just before she was diagnosed with osteosarcoma, a common cancer among children and teenagers, Angela recalled, "When you're a kid, the world is small. It barely reaches beyond your own neighborhood, your school, and your family. Cancer is just a word—something that only happens to adults."

By the age of thirty-one, Angela had survived three different kinds of cancer that altered her life physically, emotionally, and spiritually. Looking back at her prolonged battle with malignancy she observed, "It's been said so many times that the Lord works in mysterious ways. I feel I am living proof of that fact. I'm convinced that each time I became ill there was a reason for my sickness, and there were many life lessons to be learned from these experiences." Facing the prospect of death, Angela recalled that "God, who controls life, seemed to take hold and guide me to safety, leaving me with insight and a strengthened spirit that can only be understood by those who have walked in my shoes."

One of three children born to Bill and Connie, Angela was what some people would have called a "military brat." Blessed with a flaming mass of thick, curly red hair, she was fairly tall for thirteen. That was when she was diagnosed with osteosarcoma, a form of cancer that attacks first the bone, then the lungs. As a result, her right leg had to be amputated, and she underwent four subsequent operations to remove a series of recurring tumors. "This was the most dangerous of all my cancers, but it didn't seem as catastrophic as the cancers I would face as an adult. I guess that's the beauty of childhood. Nothing ever seems so terrible that life won't go on. Not even cancer."

Like a Sad Movie

Cancer brought drastic changes to Angela and her family. "It all seemed to happen so fast. Although I can recall much of my childhood cancer with great detail, it's almost as if I didn't really live it. Looking back, it's like I've been watching a sad movie about someone else's life."

The summer before she began the eighth grade, Angela had been her usual active self. She played softball and spent all her free time roller skating or bike riding with her friends. "I never did any of these things again," Angela recalled. "Although I missed them, I still have great memories of an almost perfect childhood."

The night before the first day of eighth grade, Angela and her friends were about to leave for what was to be the last of their late-night summer swims. As she changed into her swimsuit, Angela noticed that one of her hip bones looked different. She showed her mother.

Connie, a nurse, immediately sensed cause for alarm. Without letting Angela see the worry she felt, she told Angela that she would take her to the doctor the next day. And she sent Angela on her way to swim.

Memories of that night are vividly etched into Angela's mind. "I'll never forget how I felt—so full of energy and anticipation for the first day of school. We swam late into the night. Then I went to bed without a clue about what my future held."

After school the next day, Connie took Angela to a nearby clinic for X rays. It was a Monday. After she had been X-rayed, a confused radiologist "told us to come back the following day to see an orthopedic specialist. I never went back to school that year. I was admitted to the hospital the next day, a Tuesday, for more tests. I remember crying myself to sleep. It was to have been the first night of my dance lessons for the new season. I had been so excited." The instructor had chosen Angela and her best friend, Julie, to participate in a dance class with adults because she felt the two of them had the most potential. But Angela would never go for another dance lesson.

That Wednesday, after what seemed like endless X rays, the doctors told Angela's parents that she had a dislocated hip, but they would keep her in the hospital for further observation. Angela's mother did not agree with the diagnosis. She argued that if this were a dislocated hip, Angela would be unable to walk without pain or a limp. It turned out Connie was right.

Since the family lived near an army base where her father was stationed in North Carolina, they did not have the benefit of the most sophisticated medical care. But as Angela recalled, "I found out my guardian angel was working overtime. All through my life, I have found myself in situations that could have been deadly. Something or someone always happened to pull me and my family from danger. These things seem to happen when you least expect them. Often you don't understand their significance until much later. Sometimes they seem like little things. These are the things that reinforce your belief in angels, miracles, and God. They have no earthly explanation. But I call them the little things that reinforce faith and keep you going when it seems easiest to give up."

The Day of Small Things

For Angela, as for many other cancer victims as well as individuals from all walks of life, small things could seem coincidental. However, a Christian perspective recognizes that what often seems *coincidental* is in fact *providential.*

Unfortunately, it is easy to ignore or simply overlook small things in an era of summit conferences, Super Bowls, and megachurches. Yet there's a biblical principle that reminds us to look for the hand of God in what may seem less than significant. This principle is found in an Old Testament book written by a prophet named Zechariah.

Zechariah was a Levite born in Babylon, one of fifty thousand exiles who returned to the promised land of Israel to face a bleak situation. Years of spiritual apathy laced with internal conflict had stifled efforts to rebuild the temple, the center of worship in Israel. During this time, God spoke to Zechariah through a series of eight visions, one of which showed a gold lamp stand and two olive trees. This vision seemed to promise to a people whose light had just about gone out that God could provide an endless source of energy that would enable them to function as His light in a dark world.

God's message couldn't have come at a more opportune time. Discouragement was rampant as Zerubbabel the governor and the host of workers sought to complete the temple construction in the face of opposition (Ezra 4:4–5). Furthermore, though many in Israel were celebrating because of the reconstruction of the temple, many of the priests, Levites, and patriarchs who had seen the original temple wept and mourned because of the small size of this house of worship when compared to Solomon's magnificent structure (3:12–13). The thoughts of many must have paralleled the question in the minds of those who today face extended struggles with problems such as cancer: Are God's resources sufficient for the long haul?

"I felt an impending sense of doom that would not go away."

God's message, delivered by an angel to Zechariah and vividly reinforced by the vision of two olive trees, a large bowl for storing oil, plus a system of pipes to carry the oil from the storage reservoir to the seven lamps of the lamp stand, was unmistakable. An endless supply of divinely provided energy was available to enable God's people to overcome the insurmountable problems they faced.

Explaining the nature of the power available to Israel, the Lord reminded Zechariah that this was not by *internal* power (self-help) or by *external* power (the strength of others). Rather, this was "'by My Spirit,' says the Lord of hosts" (Zechariah 4:6). God's point to the prophet was clear: His divine spirit was the ultimate source of power. The need for this power was evident from the way the Lord described the problem Zerubbabel faced as a "great mountain."

Frequently, people from all walks of life refer to problems as mountains. Certainly the Israelites, attempting to rebuild their place of worship in the face of poverty and opposition, must have felt like they were struggling up the side of Mount Herman. World champion bicyclist Greg LeMond, interviewed while competing in the *Tour de France* after a particularly difficult day peddling through the French Alps, described his feelings as "like I've been shot."

Angela used similar words to describe her emotional and physical state when, as an adult, many years after her battle with osteosarcoma, she was diagnosed with breast cancer. "They found a lump the size of a large lemon in my left breast. It was like someone had shot me. Even though the radiologists and doctors told me not to worry, that I was much too young for breast cancer, I felt like the bottom of my world had fallen through. I was the most frightened I had ever been. I felt an impending sense of doom that would not go away. My life had been turned upside down, and for the first time I was scared I was going to die."

As Angela faced her second cancer diagnosis, the problem seemed insurmountable, just as with Israel in the days of Zechariah. And the questions in Angela's mind multiplied with growing frequency: *Where did this come from? How do you get cancer?* And another, even more crucial question: *How do I win this battle?* Yet Angela experienced the power of God sufficient for the mountain she faced.

The message from the Hebrew prophet was that this massive, specific obstacle, described as a great mountain, was a solvable problem because of God's character. "Who are you, O great mountain? Before Zerubbabel you shall become a plain! And he shall bring forth the capstone with shouts of 'Grace! Grace to it!'" (4:7).

This important statement contains two crucial balancing principles that have practical significance to those who face cancer and similar mountains today. First, God's power levels the problem. The cries of "Grace! Grace to it!" vividly underscore the fact that God specializes in leveling mountains in far superior fashion than our meager human resources ever could.

That is because of His excellent attributes: *omniscient*—He knows all the possibilities; *omnipotent*—He can direct circumstances in ways we can't even imagine; *all wise*—He understands the implications of every circumstance; *completely loving*—He delights in taking care of us.

The second principle is that we still have a responsibility to do what we are capable of doing. God's statement to Zerubbabel did *not* indicate that a divine crane would descend out of heaven to lower the capstone into place and finish the temple. Rather, Zerubbabel and his construction crew would be responsible to place the final stone in its proper position: "The hands of Zerubbabel have laid the foundation of this temple; His hands shall also finish it" (4:8)—that's the human responsibility factor; "Then you will know that the Lord of hosts has sent Me to you" (v. 9) reinforces the divine intervention.

Next followed a pointed reminder from God to Zerubbabel and his followers: "For who has despised the day of small things?" (v. 10). The point—one frequently underscored in Scripture—is clear, yet easily overlooked. Its implications for individuals facing obstacles like Angela experienced are enormous. *Don't despise little things.* Don't count as unimportant that which seems to be insignificant.

That message is echoed by another prophet—Micah. He wrote of an insignificant village from which would come the ultimate ruler of Israel, the Messiah (Micah 5:2). Hundreds of years later, Micah's prediction was fulfilled with the birth of Jesus Christ in Bethlehem.

Angela's Dad's Angel

Time after time God has intervened in seemingly impossible situations—sometimes using ordinary means, sometimes working in ways that are clearly supernatural. For Angela's father, Bill, it seemed that an angelic intervention had occurred years before Angela lost her leg to osteosarcoma. "It happened during an especially difficult time in the Vietnam War. It was like I was having this dream. I had returned home. The war was over. I was coming up a long row of steps—like at the Capitol building. All three of my children were there to meet me. They were cheering me on. 'You can do it, Dad. You can make it back!' Then, all of a sudden, I realized in the dream that there was something different about Angela. She only had one leg."

Jolted into wakefulness by what he had apparently seen in the dream, Bill rushed out of his tent. Within seconds, an incoming mortar shell scored a direct hit on the very tent where Bill had been sleeping, taking the lives of everyone inside. Was it an angel that had awakened Bill, like Peter centuries before? Was this some sort of divine preview of what would happen to Angela years later?

"My guardian angel must be working overtime."

Certainly Scripture indicates that angels are "ministering spirits sent forth to minister for those who will inherit salvation" (Hebrews 1:14). Looking back at the Vietnam incident, both Bill and his daughter, Angela, feel strongly that God intervened— both to save Bill's life and to help prepare him for what Angela would undergo.

Another of those seemingly "little" incidents occurred the day after Angela was misdiagnosed as having a dislocated hip. It was the incident that would lead her to say, "My guardian angel must be working overtime." A young doctor had just been transferred from Texas to the hospital in North Carolina. After examining Angela and looking at her X rays, he told Bill and Connie, "I'm convinced it's a tumor." He had just been working with another little girl who had a similar growth, an osteosarcoma, in her arm. "You simply must take her to a larger hospital—" he told Angela's parents, "one better equipped to test for and treat cancer."

That apparently chance, yet providential, encounter took place on Thursday, three days after Angela had first been taken to the clinic. By the next day the decision had been made— Connie and Angela would fly from North Carolina to Brooke Army Medical Center in San Antonio, Texas, one of the finest military medical facilities in the world.

Angela returned home from the hospital that weekend and prepared for the trip to Texas with childlike excitement. "I looked forward to the plane ride. I was excited about seeing my grandmother—she lived in San Antonio. And I felt like I was getting ready for a big adventure. Although I would miss my dad and two brothers, it would be fun to take a long trip with my mom. My parents never let on about how worried they really were."

Preparing for the trip with the excitement typical of a thirteen-year-old, Angela never once stopped to think about the gravity of her situation, or about the implications of having to go back into the hospital. But once she and her mother reached Texas, a chain of events—highs and lows like a roller coaster—began moving faster and faster.

The initial lump on Angela's hip had been located only a week before. The second week was filled with tests, plus visits with family. As Angela remembered, "A biopsy was scheduled for the end of the week, and my father flew in to be with us. The day he arrived, Dad took my cousins and me to see the Alamo and the other historical sites around San Antonio. I felt pretty strange because the doctors made me ride in a wheelchair. Everyone was beginning to treat me differently. I enjoyed the attention and the gifts, but I didn't understand why everyone was so focused on me. I just thought it was because I was visiting and would soon be going back home. But after the biopsy, the adults began to change. By now we were into the third week of this ordeal, and it wasn't fun any longer. I was tired of being special. I just wanted to go home."

A Tuesday meeting was scheduled between Angela and her parents and the chief of pediatrics. At this meeting Angela was finally told she had cancer. "It all still seems sort of surreal. I remember the doctor explaining that I had cancer, but I don't remember anything more. I asked the doctor if I would still be able to walk, and he said yes. I didn't cry, and all the adults told me how brave I was. I remember my parents saying they were proud of me. They didn't cry either."

That night volunteers from Brooke Hospital took some of the children to see the Ice Capades. Angela recalled watching the skaters, thinking it was one of the most beautiful things she had ever seen. The next morning, filled with excitement, the only thing she could talk about was ice skating. She told her parents she wanted to learn to ice skate and refused to listen when they tried to explain that there were more important things ahead for her. "I still didn't understand. I just wanted to skate. I couldn't stop talking about it. I pretended to skate around the hospital, showing my parents every move I had observed the night before. I told them I was better, and the slight limp the doctors had noticed was beginning to go away."

Angela could not understand why her parents looked at her with such sorrow when she was so happy. She felt better than ever. She was sure she would learn to ice skate. Years later Angela would discover that, by this time, Bill and Connie had already been told that her leg would have to be amputated. If she survived the extensive surgery, their best estimate was that she would live only six months longer. Alone together, Bill and Connie wept. But they never let Angela see their anguish.

An Artificial Leg

The next day Angela's favorite doctor told her they would have to take her leg. The thirteen-year-old cheerleader who wanted to be a professional dancer or ice skater, who played softball and spent all her free time roller skating or bike riding, asked if she could get an artificial leg and do everything she used to do. The doctor replied yes—but it wouldn't be the same. "She told me I would be different," Angela recalled. "I wouldn't be able to run or ride my bike. That's when I cried."

Where did Angela's cancer come from? What caused the horrible devastation, the rampaging cells that forced the removal of the right leg of this active young teenager? Over and over Angela would ask, "How did I get this cancer?"

Breast cancer affects one out of every nine women in America. It can be fatal, but it can also be beaten.

Phyllis raised the same question when she phoned our live radio talk show one night when the three authors of this book were discussing the emotional effects of cancer. Relating her story, Phyllis explained that her mother had died years before of breast cancer. It had spread through the lymph nodes to the lung.

Now an adult in her midfifties, Phyllis had just discovered a lump in her left breast. Compounding her concern was the fact that her thirty-three-year-old daughter had recently undergone a mastectomy. "I hope this lump is just a calcium deposit or a fibroid tumor," Phyllis wistfully expressed. A biopsy would be necessary to tell the doctors whether or not her tumor was malignant, whether lumpectomy, a removal of the breast tumor, or a mastectomy, surgical removal of the entire breast, would be required.

Breast cancer is extremely common in our society today. It occurs most frequently in women over fifty but also afflicts many women in their thirties and forties. Well-known singer Olivia Newton John was diagnosed with breast cancer at age forty-four. A mastectomy on her right breast was followed by intensive chemotherapy. Breast cancer affects one out of every nine women in America. It can be fatal, but it can also be beaten. Seven years after undergoing a double mastectomy, actress and singer Ann Jillian is cancer free and enjoying life after giving birth to her first child, a boy.

Angela's Breast Cancer

Like Phyllis, Olivia Newton John, and Ann Jillian, Angela didn't expect to be diagnosed with breast cancer. Since the threat of her osteosarcoma was now far behind, she felt there was less chance of her getting another cancer of any kind. "I thought I had paid my debt. I would never be sick with cancer again. I was wrong. Lightning can strike twice—but not always in the same place."

She was in her midtwenties when the lemon-sized lump was found in her left breast. "The first thing I did was go to my room and cry. I knew it would be cancer, even though statistics said I was too young even to need a mammogram." Angela's next response was to call her mother, who immediately tried to encourage and console her with the statistical unlikelihood that her tumor was malignant.

The radiologists and doctors told Angela the same thing. "Don't worry. You're much too young for breast cancer. It's probably just a benign fibrocystic disease. We should be able to take care of it easily."

But Angela felt like she had fallen through the bottom of her world. "Nobody would listen to me. I felt as if I was being patronized. It was like being a child again. But this time I wanted to be heard. I needed to be fully informed, not just told that everything would be all right."

A biopsy was scheduled for Angela. Biopsies are the only definitive way to diagnose cancer. There are four major types of biopsies: incisional, excisional, needle, and aspiration.

An *incisional biopsy* involves cutting into a tumor at the point where the tumor touches normal tissue. A portion of both tumor and normal cells is removed and compared.

An *excisional biopsy* is used when the tumor is small enough to be entirely removed. Sometimes excisional biopsy constitutes sufficient treatment for a tumor in and of itself.

A *needle biopsy* is accomplished by inserting a wide, hollow needle into a tumor in order to remove a plug of tissue for microscopic examination.

An *aspiration biopsy* utilizes a similar approach, except that a suction device is attached to the needle.

Such biopsies can determine whether or not a tumor is malignant, but they cannot reveal the degree of spread of a tumor.

The diagnosis of cancer by using a biopsy and microscopically examining tissue is referred to as a *histological diagnosis*,[1] since histology is the study of tissues. The next best approach is what is called a *cytological diagnosis,* or examination of the specific cells. The most commonly used cytological procedure is the "Pap smear," which is named after George Papanicolaou, who devised the technique in 1928. This procedure, used in diagnosing cervical cancer, involves scraping the cervix to remove cells for analysis to determine whether any are abnormal or cancerous. The tongue, esophagus, stomach, or even the air passages of the lung can also be scraped by using a small brush inserted through a scope. These cells are then put on slides, stained with dyes, and examined under a microscope.

The presence of cancer can also be determined by a number of other investigative procedures, some of which are carried out during a routine physical examination—which should be a yearly event for everyone. The annual physical exam is a thorough, systematic, progressive investigation of the body for any indications of disease or abnormality. A good checkup involves careful attention to parts of the body that are most prone to malignancy. For example, the nose and throat are visually examined, and a quick and painless examination of the larynx is done using a mirror. The lymph nodes are checked—the neck above the collarbone, the groin area, and under the arms. Special attention is paid to the breasts in women and the prostate gland in men. The examining physician will carefully push and probe the abdomen looking for any enlargement of abdominal organs, especially the spleen and liver. A careful examination of the pelvic area in women, including a Pap smear, helps detect cancers of the cervix, uterus, or ovaries. Probing the rectum with a gloved finger is an essential part of the physical for both males and females.

During the physical, a conscientious physician will ask a wide range of questions about various body functions. Frequently these parallel the American Cancer Society's list of seven early warning signals, which are referenced by the acrostic CAUTION.[2]

Change in bowel or bladder habits
A sore that does not heal
Unusual bleeding or discharge
Thickening or lump in breast or elsewhere
Indigestion or difficulty in swallowing
Obvious change in wart or mole
Nagging cough or hoarseness

Any suspicious findings on the part of the physician will lead to further tests. These usually include blood tests. Nonspecific blood tests can reveal blood abnormalities such as an elevated white cell count or an abnormality in liver function. Specific blood tests include those for so-called "tumor markers," proteins or other chemicals produced by different kinds of cancer. Bone marrow analysis is a similar procedure in which a small amount of liquid bone marrow is drawn from the breast or pelvic bone into a syringe to be examined under the microscope. Other kinds of tests are performed on bodily excretions, such as urinalysis or the hemoccult test for invisible traces of blood that may indicate the presence of a tumor or polyp in the colon.

Whenever the physical exam or lab test results indicate something suspicious, the physician will want to know just exactly what's taking place inside the body. Since there are both obvious and subtle risks to simply opening up the body and looking inside—the obvious risk of infection and surgical trauma, plus the more subtle risk of aggravating the cancer cells in a tumor growth—modern techniques of imaging can show the physician what is happening. Plain examinations, X rays, CAT scans, magnetic resonance imaging (MRI), and ultrasound are all what are termed noninvasive techniques that can help pinpoint the presence and extent of cancer.

When noninvasive imaging isn't enough, techniques such as endoscopy permit the insertion of thin telescopes to look inside body cavities through natural openings such as the nose, mouth, or urethra. Modern, flexible, fiber-optic "telescopes" actually allow for examination of the lung passages with a bronchoscope. A colonoscope allows for similar examination of the entire stomach and colon. Pieces of tissue can even be collected for biopsy purposes during the procedure. Angiography is the way to demonstrate the arterial supply to a specific area, such as the heart or a tumor.

Where Did It Come From?

All these techniques, utilized to determine the presence of cancer in Angela, Phyllis, and other patients, still don't answer the big question: Where does the cancer come from? The answer to the question "What causes cancer?" isn't a simple one. After all, the human body is a remarkable creation. With hundreds of muscles, miles of blood vessels, billions of cells, and a complex array of chemicals, the body is a tremendous reactive mechanism. As the psalmist observed centuries before Christ, we are "fearfully and wonderfully made" (Psalm 139:14).

However, whereas the body can heal itself, fight disease, grow, and survive a host of abusive factors, no body can last forever. Because of the degenerative impact of the Fall, the death process is actually present and active in every human being. God told Adam, "Of every tree of the garden you may freely eat; but of the tree of the knowledge of good and evil you shall not eat, for in the day that you eat of it you shall surely die" (Genesis 2:16–17). Since the verses that follow record that neither Adam nor Eve immediately fell dead upon eating the forbidden fruit, we understand God's pronouncement to mean that the death process, which was not present in the original perfect creation, began working in their bodies the moment they sinned.

A combination of heredity and environment seems to be the most obvious culprit when cancer comes.

Cancer provides a classic illustration of how this death process works. Although the individual who contracts cancer will, in most cases, not have committed some specific sin that brought on the cancer, it is accurate to say that every case of cancer can ultimately be traced to the tragic effects of sin on the human race.

THE GENETIC FACTOR

This raises an immediate question about genetic factors. Cancer researchers have long noted that some individuals can work for years, perhaps an entire lifetime, cancer free, despite repeated exposure to strong carcinogens such as asbestos. At the other end of the spectrum are individuals who have contracted lung cancer, for example, after only a brief exposure to asbestos. Such variation provides a strong indication of a genetic link to cancer susceptibility.

Research on the children of women exposed to DES (diethylstilbestrol) has provided another line of evidence for a genetic connection. DES, an artificial estrogen drug given during the early fifties to prevent pregnant women from miscarrying, has been linked to rare forms of vaginal cancers in the female children of women who took the drug.

Research in this area does not indicate that a person actually "inherits cancer." Rather, a predisposition to develop malignancy is what seems to be inherited.

THE ENVIRONMENTAL FACTOR

As is the case in many other disorders, a combination of heredity and environment seems to be the most obvious culprit when cancer comes. For years, research has pointed to a variety of factors in our environment whose proliferation has paralleled that of the increase of cancer. Many of these environmental factors cause changes in the DNA structure, which can somehow impair the controls the Creator has built into the process of cell reproduction and lead to the growth of cancerous cells.

DNA, deoxyribonucleic acid, discovered by James Watson and Frances Crick in 1953, is the substance at the center of every human cell. In fact, all living cells, as well as viruses and bacteria, are dependent on DNA. (Some viruses are RNA—ribonucleic acid—dependent.) Without DNA there is no life, no ability for cells to reproduce. The forty-six chromosomes of each human cell, carrying thousands upon thousands of genes, are made up of DNA. It is an incredibly complex substance— the building material of life itself!

Three out of four families in America today have been affected by cancer.

Ultraviolet light, for example, can cause changes in DNA and is thought to be responsible for most skin cancers. An increase in ultraviolet light because of depletion of the ozone layer through pollution and the use of chlorofluorocarbon (CFC) aerosol sprays has paralleled the increased rate of skin cancer being diagnosed today. Perhaps the most significant environmental factor, documented in study after study, is the carcinogenic nature of tobacco smoke. For centuries now, people from all walks of life have been smoking tobacco—using pipes, cigars, and cigarettes.

In 1981, Sir Richard Doll and Richard Peto, two pioneers in cancer epidemiology, published a landmark work entitled "The Causes of Cancer" in the *Journal of the National Cancer Institute.* Their research established diet and tobacco as the major factors in causing cancer, and ultimately cancer death. Their conclusion? "The truth seems to be that there is quite good evidence that cancer is largely an avoidable (although not necessarily a modern) disease, but with some important exceptions, [there is] frustratingly poor evidence as to exactly what are the really important ways of avoiding a reasonable percentage of today's cancers."[3]

Peto and Doll pointed out that not everything in our environment causes cancer. However, diet and tobacco are the major factors that contribute to almost two-thirds of all cancer deaths. Peto and Doll suggested that the role of heredity in cancer is probably overestimated by most people. One reason why many people view heredity as a major factor is because cancer appears in so many families. Three out of four families in America today have been affected by cancer. The family unaffected by cancer is the exception rather than the rule.

On to M.D. Anderson

In contrast to her response to the cancer she faced in childhood, Angela's diagnosis of breast cancer caused her to begin wrestling with those big questions: Where did this cancer come from? Was it caused from hereditary factors? What role did environment play? These are among the questions we frequently hear raised by those who have cancer.

Angela's doctors in Houston, where she then lived, scheduled her for breast surgery. Feeling devastated and hopeless, she cried all the way to the operating room. As the anesthesiologist began to prepare her for surgery, a nurse intervened, saying that the surgeon had decided to postpone the operation. "I had been climbing the walls," Angela recalled. "Really distraught. I was confused about why the surgery was postponed. But I was glad. My immediate thought was that the doctors had decided that my cancer was so far advanced that surgery would be in vain. But I was to find out that my guardian angel was again working overtime."

Remarkably, another doctor who had just started working at the hospital where Angela was being treated became involved in her care. He was quite familiar with breast cancer. "He told my parents there were many options available, and recommended that I go to M.D. Anderson Cancer Center here in

Houston for testing. I remember talking to my mom about how strange these coincidences were—doctors coming out of nowhere. Mom was sure these were not coincidental events but further evidence that God and His angels were looking after us. I had to agree with her. There was no other rational explanation."

So with faith renewed, Angela took her diagnosis of breast cancer to M.D. Anderson for confirmation of the diagnosis, surgery, and follow-up treatments. "Again God placed just the right person across my path," Angela recalled—"an angel of mercy." She became Angela's oncology nurse, therapist, and friend. Her name was Ginger.

Day after day during the course of her treatment, Angela would ply Ginger with questions. In return she would receive answers, plus encouragement and hope. Over the course of the six-week period, one of the major subjects of discussion was, "Where did my cancer come from? Did I inherit it?"

After all, as Angela told Ginger one day, "I have some pretty unusual things in my background genetically. I was born without quite a few of my permanent teeth—they never came in. And there were some other factors as well."

"Heredity is a factor, Angela," Ginger replied. "But its role in cancer is probably not as significant as most people think. After all, one out of three people in America will be diagnosed with cancer at some time in their life. The cancer you're fighting—breast cancer—is one of those that does seem to have a significant hereditary factor, especially where mothers and sisters in a family are diagnosed with breast cancers before menopause. Skin cancers, in families where members inherit a fair skin, and colorectal cancers that occur before the age of fifty also seem to have a pretty significant hereditary factor. But I believe the biggest factor, Angela, is the environment. Everything outside your genes. Just think about all the things we are exposed to today that contribute to cancer."

"You mean like cigarette smoke? But I don't smoke, Ginger. Never have."

"That's good, Angela. But secondhand cigarette smoke is one of the biggest culprits in exposing people to toxic chemicals. Industrial pollution and fumes from automobile exhaust are other major factors in life today. Just drive the freeways around Houston—you'll see what I mean."

"What about radiation?" Angela asked, a frown on her face.

"Sure, that's another cancer-causing factor. We're exposed to radiation all the time from the sun, not to mention radiation from X-ray equipment—even from nuclear power plants. Then there's electromagnetic radiation from high voltage power lines. Some people consider that a major factor. And radon gas, which comes naturally from the soil. Then there are toxic chemicals found in the foods we eat and the water we drink. In fact, our modern lifestyle doesn't just leave us exposed to a variety of cancer-causing agents. There are actually some that we *intentionally* consume."

Shifting position in her bed, Angela replied, "You mean like tobacco?"

"Among other things," Ginger replied, ticking off a list of items on her fingers. "We consume tobacco products. We consume high quantities of fat and protein from red meat and dairy products. Then there are large amounts of overprocessed foods, not to mention some of the preservatives used to extend the shelf life of food—or even the pesticides that find their way into both vegetables and meats. Even excessive amounts of alcohol and caffeine have been shown to cause cancer. Then there's the high-stress, Type A lifestyle many of us lead, plus unresolved emotional conflict. I read recently in one of the health magazines that up to 90 percent of cancers are caused by things we do to ourselves."

Pulling a copy of the summary of a study from her briefcase, Ginger handed it to Angela. "Take a look at this chart. You'll notice that diet at 35 percent and tobacco at 30 percent are the two most significant factors in causing cancer. Although it's not absolutely certain, it's believed that infection plays a part in 10 percent of cancers, sexual or reproductive practices in 7 percent, occupational factors in 4 percent, alcohol in 3 percent, exposure to sunshine and radiation in 3 percent, and pollution in 2 percent."

"What about food additives and industrial products?" Angela asked. "How big a factor are they?"

"They're actually included in the study." Ginger turned a page. "You'll notice they're on this other chart. But the study indicates that they are the identifiable cause in less than 1 percent of cancer deaths."

Causes of Cancer Deaths By Percentage

Diet	35%
Tobacco	30%
Infection	10%
Sexual or reproductive practices	7%
Occupational factors	4%
Alcohol	3%
Exposure to sunshine and radiation	3%
Pollution	2%
Food additives	less than 1%
Industrial products	less than 1%

Reflecting back over her experience when diagnosed with osteosarcoma as a child, Angela thought about one fear she had entertained from time to time, one she had also observed in others. "I remember becoming aware that some people were afraid they could catch cancer from me. Some of my friends, for example, seemed hesitant to get around me. Would that be borne out by the 10 percent of cancers in this study caused by infections?"

Ginger shook her head. "My years here at M.D. Anderson have convinced me that cancer isn't caught. The nurses, doctors, and other people who work with cancer patients day after day don't catch cancer. If that were the case, you'd see staff members here dropping like flies. I think what this study indicates is that you can't get cancer from touching a person like you can catch other things. But it is true that you can catch certain infections from cancer patients or from others, like HIV or Hepatitis B, that can lead to certain forms of cancer."

"It seems like that's something we ought to let children know."

"No doubt about it. We especially need to encourage and reassure children that they can't catch cancer from a parent or a friend."

"Any other misconceptions about things that cause cancer?" Angela wondered, seizing the opportunity to increase her knowledge.

"Well, I've known of people who mistakenly felt that performing surgery actually caused cancer—that a swelling or lump didn't become malignant until it was actually cut open. There is no evidence to back up that idea—or the notion that a blow to your body or some other kind of trauma can cause cancer. Sometimes people think that's the case when what has actually happened is that a blow or trauma has called attention to a preexisting cancerous lump."

"What about a chronic irritation, such as a poorly fitting denture?"

"The studies I've read," Ginger replied, "indicate that chronic irritation is more of a by-product of many cancer-causing substances. However, I believe there are occasions when chronic irritations, such as a poorly fitting denture, can lead to the development of a cancer.

Tobacco use [is] responsible for 30 percent of all cancer deaths, 30 percent of all heart disease deaths, and 80 percent of all chronic lung disease deaths.

"The major factor influencing the development of nine of the ten leading cancers in the United States is dietary practices. That's why both the American Cancer Society and the National Cancer Institute have issued dietary recommendations to try to reduce the risk of cancer. Diet, for example, accounts for 90 percent of the risk for bowel cancer, 50 percent for breast cancer, and 20 percent for lung cancer. That's why the National Academy of Sciences in its report *Diet, Nutrition and Cancer* concluded that by changing dietary practices, the American public could reduce its incidence of cancer by approximately one-third."[4]

In the pivotal 1982 report Ginger mentioned to Angela, dietary guidelines strongly recommended that fat intake be reduced and consumption of fresh fruits, vegetables, and whole grains be increased. A follow-up study urged Americans to reduce their fat intake to less than 30 percent of total calories, while increasing their dietary fiber to 20 to 30 grams per day and consuming more fresh fruits and vegetables, especially those high in vitamins A and C.

Tobacco and Cancer

In 1979, Surgeon General J. B. Richmond issued the landmark ruling that, "Cigarette smoking is clearly the largest, single preventable cause of illness and premature death in the United States." Studies released by his office pointed to tobacco use as responsible for 30 percent of all cancer deaths, 30 percent of all heart disease deaths, and 80 percent of all chronic lung disease deaths.

Angela and Ginger discussed the smoke factor a few days after their conversation about diet and cancer. "Did you know that tobacco causes more than 350,000 deaths per year in the United States?" Ginger asked Angela. "That may not sound like a huge number, but it's the equivalent of three fully loaded jumbo jet liners crashing—killing everyone on board—every single day, over a year's time."

"Incredible! You'd think with information like that everybody would quit smoking."

"Plenty of people would like to. But it's a terribly addictive habit. And the real tragedy is the effect on 'secondhand smokers'—like children and spouses of smokers, and fellow workers. They are at extremely high risk because of exposure to the hundreds of chemicals found in tobacco smoke."

"What kinds of chemicals?" Angela asked. "I guess I usually just thought of smoke as containing nicotine."

"That's a major culprit, all right. I read the other day that the amount of nicotine found in one cigarette can be lethal to a child. But cigarette smoke also contains carbon monoxide, tar, ammonia, formaldehyde, creosote, arsenic, and lead, among other chemicals. I read that nicotine and carbon monoxide are the big factors in cardiovascular diseases, but tar is the major cancer-causing agent in tobacco. It's the primary factor in lung cancer, which causes about a fourth of all cancer deaths." Pulling another report from her briefcase, Ginger studied it for a moment, then looked back up at Angela. "It says here that more than 135,000 people die from lung cancer in America each year. And 83 percent of lung cancer is caused by cigarette smoking."

Ginger slipped the report back into her briefcase. "Lung cancer kills almost nine out of every ten people diagnosed with it within five years—and there's no effective method of early detection. Back in the early eighties, we noticed an epidemic of lung cancer among women who continued to smoke even after the surgeon general's warnings were issued."

"Probably because of all those ads that made it look cool for women to smoke," Angela mused.

"I suspect so. That's about the time lung cancer overtook breast cancer as the leading cause of cancer death in women."

"Doesn't lung cancer affect only smokers?"

"No way!" Ginger replied. "I read recently that exposure to secondary cigarette smoke increases the incidence of lung cancer in nonsmokers by as much as 30 percent. Overall, the figures I read indicate that secondary smoking accounts for up to five thousand deaths per year."

"I guess I was wondering more about things like smoke-less tobacco. Does that cut out the risk of cancer?"

"That's a very common misconception. I think some people have turned to smokeless tobacco in the belief that by not inhaling they will be protected from cancer. But smokeless tobacco has been shown to be the culprit in cancers of the lip, mouth, lung, and throat. Plus it contributes to tooth decay, gum disease, and bad breath."

A Third Malignancy

One day during the months Angela spent at M.D. Anderson being treated for breast cancer, she discovered another lump on her body, located on her right biceps. Angela insisted that the doctors check it out. At first it seemed that no one took it seriously—one doctor dismissed it as a harmless fibrous tumor. Angela recalls him "telling me that it was highly unlikely that I had two cancers at the same time—that I was probably just getting paranoid."

The following week, Angela showed the lump to Ginger, who immediately reinforced Angela's request to have the lump carefully checked out. At this point the doctor agreed, ordering a simple needle biopsy. Sure enough, the suspicious mass turned out to be malignant leiomyosarcoma. When surgery was performed for her breast cancer, the lump in her right arm was removed as well.

In our conversations with numerous cancer patients, we have discovered that the question "How did I get cancer?" is extremely common, following just behind, "Will I be able to get over it?" and "Will I die of it?" Yet we are convinced that, for anyone diagnosed with cancer, the most important question is not how did you get it, but what cancer do you have. And what treatment do you need? Quick and early diagnosis followed by prompt, appropriate treatment is essential. Another essential is the kind of faith Angela developed—an active, strong faith in God based on His ability to work in the "small things" as well as the "big things" in diagnosis and treatment. Active faith and the best medical care are the key factors in successfully facing the threat of cancer.

5

CANCER AND THE PHYSICAL

Tom* came storming into the reception area of Dr. Blake's office, muttering under his breath about poorly timed rain showers. Raindrops beaded on his leather jacket as rivulets dripped from the brim of his ten-gallon hat.

"Sorry about all the water," he said as he wiped his size 13 cowboy boots on the doormat, removed his hat and jacket, then walked over to the receptionist to check in.

"Guess the doc's gonna tell me more about this cancer business today," he said, a smile touching the corners of his leathery face. He wore a no-frills, plaid Western shirt atop worn Levi 501 denim jeans, held up by a wide belt with a massive bronze buckle in the shape—and approximately the size—of the state of Texas.

In a matter of minutes, Tom was seated in a conference room just down the hall from the treatment room where he had first been confronted with the possibility that he had prostate cancer. "So what do you think about this weather, Doc?" Tom began somewhat nervously as Dr. Blake entered the room. "It's a real frog strangler out there, isn't it? Keep this up, we'll have to build an ark or something."

* Tom's story began in chapter 1.

Dr. Blake smiled, picked up a manila folder from his desk, opened it, and began glancing through the charts. "Just as I suspected, Tom—an adenocarcinoma of the prostate, poorly differentiated—a T-3 N-2 M-2. Pretty serious stuff, Tom. We need to get right to work on a plan to lick this thing."

"What do you mean, get right to work, Doc? I've already been worked over pretty good! That kid that stuck that needle in me yesterday—that's a pretty delicate place to stick a needle. I mean, I consider myself a pretty tough guy and all that. Had a few times I took someone to fist city out in the oil fields. And I've had needles stuck in me before, but . . . but, hey! Come on! Then they put me in that tunnel, and I just about freaked out. What did you call that thing? A CAT scan? I didn't see any cats in there."

Dr. Blake noticed the twinkle in Tom's eye. "You're just giving me a hard time, aren't you, Tom?"

"Not a chance, Doc. Do I look like the kind of guy who would give a poor cancer doc a hard time? What was that fancy term you used? Uncle Ologist?"

Dr. Blake chuckled aloud as he corrected his patient. "Oncologist, Tom. Oncologist." Moving from his desk to a white acrylic marker board, the slim physician picked up the red marker and wrote the word at the top of his board. "That's the kind of doctor I am—a doctor who specializes in treating tumors. In fact, that's what the word comes from."

He drew a line between the second O and the first L in *oncologist.* "The Latin word *onco* actually means 'tumor.' That's what cancer is—it's a tumor, a growth."

"Slow down, Doc. I don't even speak pig Latin. And what about all those numbers you were mumbling earlier? T-2, C-4. Sounds like something Warren Moon would call in a huddle— some kind of pass play. But it sounds all Greek to me—or maybe Latin. I know you're a busy man, Doc, but if you guys are gonna work me over to help me beat this cancer, I need to know what's going on. That's my approach in the oil business —I want to know everything I can about everything. Now I don't want to become a doctor myself or anything. But I'd sure like you to fill me in on what's happened to me and what you and these other medical people are gonna do about it."

Glancing at his watch, Dr. Blake said, "Well, Tom, your timing couldn't be better. You're the last patient I'm supposed to see today. And I'm actually running a little bit ahead of schedule. Tell you what, if you'd like a cup of coffee, I'll see if we can't give you a crash course in what's going on with your body and what we hope to do about it. Care for a cup?"

"Sure," Tom replied, stretching his massive six-foot-five-inch frame.

"How do you take it?"

"Black—I don't put any poisons in it. I hear sugar and cream both cause cancer," Tom said with a wink.

Dr. Blake pressed a button on his intercom. "Julie, could you please get us a couple cups of coffee? The usual in mine, black for Tom." He turned to Tom. "You see, cancer doctors are immune to cancer causing agents. And if you believe that, I have some underwater real estate I'd like to interest you in purchasing."

The two men chuckled as Dr. Blake walked around to the front of his desk, pushed the stack of books back toward the center, and perched himself on the edge. "First off, Tom, like I told you before, cancer isn't a single disease—there are probably more than a hundred different forms of cancer. But *every* cancer is a tumor. All tumors aren't cancerous, but every cancer is a tumor."

"Hold the phone, Doc. That just doesn't make sense. Every cancer is a tumor, but every tumor isn't a cancer?"

"Let me explain, Tom. You see, there are *malignant* tumors—that's the cancerous kind—and then there are the ones we refer to as *benign.* See that big mole on your left wrist? That's a form of benign tumor. A malignant tumor, on the other hand, is a pretty dangerous thing. A benign tumor may be something you're concerned about because of your looks—a lot of women are more concerned about them than men—but a malignant tumor is a source of concern for anybody."

"So how do you tell the difference, Doc?" Tom asked, leaning forward in the chair.

"Let me give you a two-part answer to that. A simple answer, plus a little background. First, malignant tumors are invasive. That is, they have the ability to invade other parts of the body. They are made up of cells that have changed so that they don't have the normal external wall that the cells in a benign tumor have—or for that matter, normal cells period." Dr. Blake walked to the marker board and drew a circle. "This represents the external wall of a cell from a benign tumor. As you can see, it has a clear-cut boundary—you can tell precisely where the tumor ends."

Dr. Blake shaded the edges of the external wall he had drawn with his finger. "This represents the external wall of a cell from a malignant tumor. Because it doesn't have a definite boundary, it can invade surrounding tissues and actually destroy them. In fact, little chunks of malignant cells can actually break off from a tumor and travel through the body like seeds. They land in other tissues, put down roots, and start additional cancerous growth."

Cancer is invasive.

"You make these things sound like bands of outlaws, Doc—like those gangs in some of the Western novels I like to read. They just sort of run around wreaking havoc till somebody finally comes along who can outshoot 'em."

"That's actually a fairly accurate description of our fight against cancer, Tom," Dr. Blake said, nodding. "In fact, you might call some of the treatments we use today 'Gunfight at the O.K. Corral.'"

A Nightmare of Metastasis

What Tom was learning during his discussion with Dr. Blake is one of the most important principles about the physical characteristics of the disease we are considering: *Cancer is invasive.*

As explained in chapter 4, many factors are at work on the cells in the bodies we carry through life. Some are external, such as tobacco and tobacco smoke, industrial agents, or toxic substances. Some are more internal—for example, the high-fat, low-fiber diets that are so common today. Others include sexual practices, particularly those involving sexually transmitted viruses. Even medical treatments (such as X rays) or hormones (such as DES) or excessive exposure to sunlight can initiate cancer. So how does a tumor develop within the human body? Let's go back to the conversation between Tom and Dr. Blake to find out.

"So how long has this malignant stuff been in me, Doc? You've already told me you can't say for sure what gave it to me."

"To be honest, Tom, I don't know for sure. But I suspect it could have been as long as ten, twenty, even thirty years."

"I quit smoking a few years ago, Doc. Think smoking's what caused it?"

"Smoking doesn't seem to be a factor in prostate cancer, although smoking is certainly the primary cause of lung cancer and a lot of other cancers today. And I don't know if you've been exposed to radiation at work, but, generally speaking, prostate cancer isn't caused by radiation. The most common factors I've seen in patients with the kind of cancer you have are a high level of fat in the diet, an increased number of sexual partners, and venereal disease."

"Hey, Doc. You're not gonna start meddling in my personal life, are you?" Tom asked, a rather stern look on his face. "I mean, I'm not the kind of hard livin' guy I used to be."

The doctor shook his head. "I'm not here to condemn you, Tom, just to treat you."

"More like persecute me! Having that guy stick that needle in me, putting me inside that machine!"

Not sure whether his patient was kidding or serious at this point, Dr. Blake decided to play it safe. "We had to do that needle biopsy right at that spot. I know it's delicate. But that's the only way we can tell for sure about the tumor. The CAT scan, better yet the MRI scan, is a fancy, three-dimensional imaging, or picture, process. It works well for prostate cancer— helps us find out to what extent it has spread. I suspect we may have to do some more biopsies on some of your lymph nodes from the looks of this report."

"I don't want to think about that right now, Doc. Let's get back to how this thing started."

"Actually, it probably started with a multiple hit on a single cell."

Dr. Blake turned back to his board and wrote two words:

SINGLE

CELL

Next he drew a small circle, then wrote two more words:

MULTIPLE
HIT

"There are actually several theories about how cancer starts, but most of the specialists I respect see it happening this way: Imagine that you could put your body under an incredibly powerful microscope. You'd see millions of cells—billions would probably be more accurate. Every one of these cells has twenty-three pairs of chromosomes."

"Pretty small, these cells—right?"

"Small all right, but not the smallest part of the body. In fact, there could be anywhere from fifty- to one-hundred-thousand genes in every human cell, located along the chromosomes. But, out of that huge number, there are probably about a hundred genes in each cell that regulate the way that cell grows or divides. Now most of the cells in our body divide—that's normal. There are periods when the division and growth are very rapid—for example, when a baby is in its mother's womb, and between childhood and the teenage years."

Tom grinned, understanding. "Yeah, that's what happened to my son. He shot up from five to six feet almost overnight. Put on about forty pounds. Do you suppose some of his genes went haywire?"

"Probably not," Dr. Blake replied. "But sometimes a few genes will take a *hit* from some of the things we call carcinogens—those are cancer-causing factors."

"Sort of like bullets, eh, Doc?" Tom inquired, rubbing his chin. "I was in some fire fights during the Korean War. Got hit by shrapnel a couple of times. Wound up with a purple heart."

"Well, that's sort of what happens," Dr. Blake said. "Some scientists think viruses of different kinds cause the hits on genes that prompt a normal cell to change into a malignant cell. Most of the research literature I've been reading lately seems to indicate that all cancers come from at least two or more hits, or changes, to the genes in a given cell. It's like these hits sort of build up over time, until eventually a breaking point is reached and a cell becomes malignant."

Dr. Blake drew a dark, shaded circle on his board. Beneath this he drew a larger, irregularly shaped circle. "What happens after this change in the cell—we call it a mutation—is that the cell begins to multiply rapidly. The single abnormal cell becomes two abnormal cells, then four. Researchers refer to these as doubling times. Some fast-growing cancers may double in a matter of weeks. Others take months. For example, in the case of your cancer, it could have taken five years before the doubling process happened twenty times."

The risk of developing cancer actually depends on three major factors: who you are, where you live, and how you live.

"So that's how big the tumor was when you found it, Doc?"

"No. Actually at that point your tumor was probably only the size of a pinhead. There's no way you could feel it at that size or even spot it by a scan, even though it would have contained a million cells. This is what we call the *silent period* of cancer growth. Usually the doubling process has to happen thirty times or more before we can feel a lump or experience pain."

"Or have trouble going to the bathroom?" Tom asked.

"Exactly. But your problem, Tom, is that you didn't come in when you first started noticing the symptoms," Dr. Blake gently chided.

"So how come these cells start spreading, and other cells don't?"

"Quite frankly, Tom, we don't fully understand. We just know that the Creator designed all cells with a boundary and a built-in code to tell them when to stop. But different factors—like smoke, X rays—the things we call initiators—finally cause the cells to change to the point where they just go out of control. Just like some of those gangs in the Westerns you read.

"By the way, you'll be interested to know that there are certain things we call *promoters*, things that actually enhance the development of cancer cells. Alcohol, for example, promotes the growth of cancers of the head, neck, and liver. And stress can actually weaken the immune system, making us more susceptible to cancer."

"What about heredity?" Tom asked. "My dad never had cancer."

"Well, actually, heredity can be a factor. Just the other day I was reading an article that suggested that the risk of developing cancer actually depends on three major factors:[1] who you are, where you live, and how you live."

Turning to the blackboard he wrote three words to the right of his diagram:

GENETICS

ENVIRONMENT

LIFESTYLE

"Even though your dad didn't have cancer, you may have inherited some genetic tendencies from him that made you more susceptible. Your environment—living and working in an atmosphere where you are exposed to cancer-causing agents can put you at risk. And personal lifestyle choices—like smoking, high-fat, low-fiber diet, and sexual practices—can increase that risk."

"So does cancer usually start in several places in the body, or just one?"

"Cancer almost always starts at a single site. In fact, we usually label the cancer by the site where it starts, because cancers that start, for example, in the liver will have different traits than those that start in the bone or bloodstream."

Tom shifted his massive frame. "Tell me more about how these cells spread."

"Sure," Dr. Blake replied. "Usually, small clumps of cancer cells break off from the original tumor and are carried to other parts of the body. Sometimes this happens by direct extension. In other words, the tumor itself actually invades the organs or tissue right next to it. Sometimes tumors develop roots, which burrow into surrounding tissue."

"Sort of like a cypress tree?"

"That's a good example. Another way cancer can be spread is through the blood supply. After all, tumors require blood to grow, just like normal cells. Pieces of the tumor may penetrate the walls of blood vessels and be carried by the bloodstream to various other organs in the body."

Tom shuddered visibly. "Boy, that's a scary thought, Doc."

"Fortunately the process works a lot like seeds that blow off plants. A lot more of them just land and die than take root and start growing. Then there's another system in the body that's particularly susceptible to spreading cancer. It's called the lymphatic system."

Grinning, Tom interrupted. "Oh, you mean the system that causes a person to limp?"

"Not exactly. You see, usually when we think of the blood supply, we think of arteries that carry blood to the various organs in the body, like the brain, and veins that return the blood to the heart to replenish it with oxygen. This other system—the lymphatic system—is sort of like the body's sewage system. It's a system of tiny vessels—we call them *lymphatics.*"

"Sort of the opposite of *emphatics*?"

Dr. Blake chuckled. "Lymphatics carry a clear liquid called *lymph.* It drains away infectious material and other toxins from various parts of the body. Now, located along these vessels are what we call *lymph nodes,* which trap these toxic materials. The tonsils are a good example of lymphatic tissue."

The TNM system is one of several systems used by oncologists to classify the size and stage of a variety of tumors.

"Yeah," Tom replied. "When I was a kid I used to have tonsillitis. I think they took out everybody else's tonsils in my class when I was in school. But I still have mine."

"They used to take everybody's tonsils out. In fact, there was a time when they didn't think there was any use for tonsils. But the tonsils actually help with the job of trapping bacteria, preventing a lot of infection from getting into your body.

"With your background in the oil fields, Tom, you could probably visualize these lymph glands as pipelines carrying away toxic waste from a refinery. The lymph nodes would be the filtering and pumping stations along the way. Unfortunately, when cancer cells get into the system, they often spread from station to station, infecting each station as they go."

The Spread of Cancer

At this early point in Tom's treatment, he wasn't yet aware of the extent of metastasis of his particular cancer. Tom had refused for months—even years—to go to the doctor. When he finally went, it was discovered that the cancer had spread from his prostate, where it began, into nearby lymph nodes and bone tissue, and even up his back.

That's why Dr. Blake referred to his particular cancer as a T-3 N-2 M-2. The TNM system is one of several systems used by oncologists to classify the size and stage of a variety of tumors. Whenever a biopsy is performed, each tumor is given a specific rating in simplified form.

A T-0 rating indicates a tumor small enough to be completely removed by the biopsy through which the diagnosis was made. Needless to say, this is quite rare. T-1, T-2, and T-3 tumors would be progressively larger in size. By the time a T-4 rating is reached, the tumor may have spread into surrounding tissues.

The N-rating indicates the degree of involvement of nearby lymph nodes. N-0 indicates lymph nodes that are free of cancer cells. The higher the N-rating, the greater the involvement of cancer cells in the nearby lymph nodes.

The M classification refers to metastasis, or spread of the cancer to form distant tumors. An M-0 rating indicates no metastasis; M-1 or higher indicates evidence of metastasis.

This is actually an oversimplification because various stages of cancer have different classifications, and there are variations for each basic classification.

A second basic way of classifying tumors is referred to as *staging*. A Stage One cancer is generally small and has not spread beyond its original site of growth. Stage One cancers are generally considered highly curable, frequently by surgery alone. Some doctors refer to this as *carcinoma in situ*; still other doctors refer to *carcinoma in situ* as a precursor to Stage One cancer.

By Stage Two, the cancer has begun to spread through and even beyond the organ where it began. Traces of it may be found in nearby lymph nodes. Belinda, a forty-three-year-old bank executive and mother of two, was diagnosed with breast cancer classified as T-2 N-1 M-0—a one inch-diameter lesion removed from the breast, with some evidence of spread to lymph nodes in the armpit but no indication of further metastasis.

Stage Three cancer has spread into adjacent tissues and has definitely invaded the adjacent lymph nodes. The prognosis is not as good as the first two stages, although a cure is still possible. Tom's cancer would ultimately be labeled as Stage Three.

Stage Four cancer has definite evidence of metastasizing. Jessica's initial diagnosis (chapter 3) was a Stage Four cancer with involvement from the arm into the lymph nodes and the lung. Those who are diagnosed with Stage Four cancer are given little chance of survival. However, there are notable exceptions, both in terms of life expectancy and the accuracy of prognosis.

There is a third type of classification of tumors: well-differentiated and undifferentiated. When a pathologist examines a slide of tissue from a well-differentiated cancer of the pancreas, he is able to tell that he is looking at pancreatic tissue, even though it is malignant and differs from normal pancreas tissue. It has that pancreatic look, even though it is obviously abnormal.

On the other hand, undifferentiated tumors often don't look like any specific tissue at all. Pathologists often describe them as looking *primitive* or *immature.* Sometimes these classifications are referred to as *high-grade* (undifferentiated) or *low-grade* (well-differentiated). High-grade tumors tend to grow more rapidly and aggressively, whereas low-grade tumors consist of more mature cells and are more slow growing. Such information is extremely useful to the oncologist in determining both the timing and the extent of treatment needed.

For example, when oncologists at M.D. Anderson Cancer Center in Houston examined pictures of slides from the biopsies taken from Richard Block's lung (story in chapter 1), they determined the presence of an extremely high-grade tumor. Action was required immediately. He wasn't even given the option of taking a weekend off before treatment began. On the other hand, Richard's friend Gerald's diagnosis of skin cancer indicated a low-grade tumor, well-differentiated and slow growing. Although surgery needed to be scheduled, it didn't have to take place immediately.

Kinds of Tumors

Dr. Blake paused in his conversation with Tom. "Any questions about what we've talked about so far?"

"Yeah. My administrative assistant told me that there's some kinds of cancers that are better to have than others. I don't remember what she said, but maybe you can help me figure it out. Do I have the good kind?"

"Well, I'm not sure I'd call it the *good* kind. The kind of tumor you have is called a *carcinoma.*"

"Named after Johnny Carson, I suppose. Probably caused from too much time listening to late-night television talk show monologues."

"Close, but not quite," Dr. Blake replied with a grin. "Your spelling is off just a little bit." Turning to the board, he erased one section of what he had drawn, then wrote *carcinoma.*

"These are tumors that usually develop on the skin or on internal organs and surfaces—we call them the *epithelium.* Usually these tumors develop in an organ that secretes something. For example, the lungs secrete mucous, the skin perspiration. The pancreas secretes digestive juices. And the prostate secretes the fluid that makes us men."

Tom ran his rugged fingers through his hair and furrowed his brow. "When you first told me about this, Doc, you had some other word tacked on the front end of that carcinoma business."

Dr. Blake nodded. "I referred to it as an *adeno*carcinoma. That simply meant it was a tumor that originated in an organ that is glandular in nature. There are some other terms you've probably heard before. For example, *melanoma* would be cancer of the cells that give the skin its color. There are a couple of other kinds of tumors—just so you'll know. *Sarcomas* develop in bones, muscles, nerves, or tendons—connective tissues. They can even develop in blood vessels."

"So could they develop in the same place where there's a carcinoma?"

"Good question, Tom. In fact, that's not too unusual. I saw a case like that just last week. A man had a carcinoma develop in the pancreas, and another tumor in the wall of a blood vessel in the pancreas. It was a sarcoma."

"I guess you could put them under the microscope and tell the difference."

"You could—and often you need to take into account the *kind* of tumor you're dealing with when you devise a treatment plan.

"There's one other category, Tom. *Lymphomas* and *leukemias* usually develop in the lymph glands. One of the most common of these is called Hodgkin's Disease. Almost all these kinds of cancers are either referred to as Hodgkin's or non-Hodgkin's lymphomas. Leukemia is a cancer of the white blood cells."

"Pretty complicated stuff, Doc—takes a lot more schooling to understand this stuff than what you need to drill for oil."

"Right, Tom. If I've answered most of your questions, let me take a little time to go over your treatment plan."

After Dr. Blake had detailed a plan for Tom that included surgery to remove the tumor-infested prostate gland followed by both radiotherapy and chemotherapy, Tom raised another question. "I know you wouldn't let me do this, Doc, but suppose we just decided not to do anything about this cancer? Just let it go, hope it would heal itself. What do you suppose would happen? Would it kill me?"

Dr. Blake's response was careful, slow, and measured. "I'm glad you're not thinking seriously about that approach, Tom. Quite frankly, yes, I think it would ultimately kill you. But don't ask me how long it would take. I just know that this kind of cancer—when it's developed to the level of yours—is a pretty serious matter."

Kinds of Cancerous Tumors

Carcinoma	A tumor that develops on the skin or in internal organs
Sarcoma	A tumor that develops in bones, muscles, nerves, or tendons
Melanoma	A tumor that develops in certain skin cells
Lymphoma	A tumor that develops in the lymph glands
Leukemia	Tumors that develop in the white blood cells

"So what do cancer patients die of, Doc?" Tom blurted out, obviously uneasy at this point in the interview.

He's probably been thinking this for quite some time, Dr. Blake thought as he responded. "Several things, Tom. The first of these is called *cachexia.*"

Walking over to his marker board, the doctor printed the word in the upper left-hand corner, away from his other writing. "Let me explain what I mean. When cancer grows in a human body, it causes profound changes in the organs themselves and in the way they function. Some of this is caused by the cancer itself and some by the body's attempt to repair the damage the cancer does.

"We don't understand a lot about cachexia. But we know what it looks like. You've probably seen patients with terminal cancer who've looked chronically ill. Their skin is pale, their bodies wasted away. They seem apathetic. In fact, the term 'wasting away' is probably the best way I know to describe it."

Tom nodded. "That must have been what happened to my aunt. She started off with some kind of cancer of the female organs. But when they operated on her, they opened her up and just sewed her back together. Said the cancer had spread all through her body. I went to see her in the hospital. Wasn't a pleasant sight. In fact, I couldn't stand to go back to see her again. She just shriveled up into nothing. She'd even broken a bone while she was taking a bath."

"Yes, that's one of several things that can happen in cachexia," Dr. Blake replied solicitously, stroking his cheek with the index finger of his right hand. "There are a number of other things that cause death. Sometimes the cancer creates an obstruction—just the sheer size of the tumor—or it may cause the organ where it's growing to fail. Or the cancer, plus the body's attempt to fight it off, may open the body to a secondary infection. There are a lot of ways cancer can kill you.*

"But there are a lot of ways to survive cancer, Tom. That's what I want to focus on with the rest of our time. We've put a plan together that can help you lick this thing. Your surgery has been scheduled. We'll follow that up with radiotherapy, then with chemotherapy. You'll have oncology nurses working with you on the chemo, nutritionists helping you revamp your diet, and a physical therapist to help keep you in physical shape.

"And I'll be the quarterback of the team. So if you have any questions, especially any that the other individuals on the team can't answer, let me know. I've seen a lot of people with the kind of cancer you have, Tom. Quite frankly, it's not a sure thing. But I've seen a lot of them get well. It wasn't easy. Took a lot of work, both on the part of the team and on the patient's part. That means you."

Tom shuffled his feet nervously. "I've always been a hard worker, Doc. Worked hard at whatever I did. Worked hard in the oil fields. Ran my business hard. Pushed the people hard I worked with. But never harder than I pushed myself."

"That'll stand you in good stead now, Tom. We both have a lot of work ahead of us—a real fight. But I'm convinced that if we tackle this thing the way I want us to, you'll make it. One other factor I want to mention to you. That's the will to live. You mentioned fighting in the Korean War. There've been a lot of studies of prisoners of war: Victor Frankl, prisoners from Germany in World War II, and people like General Jim Stockdale in Vietnam."

"Yeah, I remember him. He's the guy who ran on the presidential ticket with Ross Perot. Didn't they hold him prisoner over there for about five or six years?"

"Six, I believe it was. But the main thing he had going for him was that he had the will to live. I'm convinced—and my colleagues at M.D. Anderson are as well—that this is probably the key ingredient that you and the other patients supply. We can provide chemotherapy, surgery, all the rest. But you have to choose to live—and then keep working at it."

* This will be dealt with in greater detail in chapter 10.

"I really wanna make it, Doc," Tom replied softly. "But I'll admit, it's scary. You said this thing is pretty far along. S'pose it's terminal?"

"Let me make some suggestions, Tom," Dr. Blake replied quickly. "One needs to be careful about linking that word *terminal* to cancer. I heard you use it a bit ago, when you were talking about your aunt. These days, we're trying to approach cancer as more of a chronic disease than as a terminal one. *Chronic* means it's long term—you usually don't beat it overnight. But that's sure different from fatal.

Patients who actively participate in their recuperation rather than just submit to treatments are the ones most likely to survive cancer.

"Another thing—you'll need all the support and encouragement you can get. That means your family, your friends, fellow workers, your pastor—and others who are close to you."

"Are you sure about that, Doc?" Tom asked, scowling. "I'm sort of a self-made person. I sure don't want to involve my kids or ask them for help. Or the people I work with."

"I want to challenge you to change your thinking on this one, Tom," Dr. Blake replied firmly. "You're going to need all the help you can get. But your personal initiative will help you on my final suggestion. You need to become what we refer to as your own 'patient advocate.' Get involved in the process. I've found that patients who actively participate in their recuperation rather than just submit to treatments are the ones most likely to survive cancer."

Getting Involved in Your Treatment

We are convinced that Dr. Blake's advice to Tom was right on target. We strongly recommend that anyone who has been diagnosed with cancer implement the following suggestions for communicating effectively with his oncologist and health-care team.

1 *Focus on communicating.* Your doctor needs to know what's going on in your life. Have you been losing weight? Suffering from diarrhea? Developing sores in your mouth? What is different since you last saw the doctor? Doctors are like football coaches or politicians—they're always trying to anticipate what the opposition will do next. As the patient, you are in the best position to help them develop and fine-tune the most effective game plan. So be sure to give the clearest, most detailed answers you can. Don't hold back anything—especially not something that could be significant—such as blood in your urine or stool, or another lump.

2 *Keep a notebook.* Sometimes it's most helpful to jot down your experiences and symptoms, so as to be prepared. Write down any questions you want to ask the doctor before each visit. Make quick notes of his answers. Sometimes using a tape recorder to record the doctor's responses to your questions— always with his permission—can be a useful means for securing information without taking up more of your physician's limited time.

3 *Don't hesitate to ask, but prioritize your questions.* Sometimes patients, obsessively concerned with their well-being, give a lengthy list of questions to the doctor, some of which are far more relevant than others. Unless you try to limit your questions to those that are most essential, and prioritize them, you stand the chance of not getting the explanations that may help you play an active role in your own treatment. At times patients may want to talk about a series of minor problems as a way of saying, "I'm really afraid," without coming out and saying so. Make sure you focus on major issues—nausea, swelling, weight changes—rather than things that are of less significance.

4 *Be cooperative.* Sometimes a lack of cooperation with the doctor stems from anxiety or fear. Sometimes it's simply the anger stage in the grief process. Every doctor who has treated cancer has probably run into patients who are either passively or actively uncooperative. This problem can range from minor matters, such as refusing to undress for an examination, to postponing important blood tests or even surgical procedures. Remember, when you refuse to cooperate with your doctor, you're not hurting him or her. You're hurting only yourself.

The patient with the greatest chance of succeeding against cancer is the patient who cooperates with his or her physician and
treatment team.

6

CANCER AND THE EMOTIONAL

Candy seemed to be the last person you'd ever associate with strong emotions such as fear, anxiety, or anger. Yet sitting in the spacious den of her home, overlooking a forest just south of Birmingham, Alabama, Candy Wood admitted that she had been afraid and anxious and intensely angry.

The reason? Candy had a most unusual cancer—an osteosarcoma rising from the base of her skull to the sinus cavity behind her right eye. According to Dr. Edward Creagan, professor of medical oncology at the Mayo Medical School and consultant to the Mayo Clinic, Candy's tumor was "in such a delicate location that relatively few surgeons, even on a global scale, would ever attempt to surgically remove this neoplasm."

As Candy perched her slender frame on a comfortable couch, she described her cancer experience while glancing occasionally at the colorful leaves swept by the chilly, autumn wind across her patio. She did not seem to be either fearful or angry. But by her own admission, she had been.

It Started with Pain

According to Candy, it all started with what seemed to be persistent sinus pain. "I went to nine different ear, nose, and throat doctors because I just couldn't seem to get over these terrible headaches. I was popping Tylenol like Sweet Tarts. But I figured my problem had to be sinuses. After all, I had a lot of sinus drainage. And living in Birmingham, most everyone I knew had sinus problems or allergies."

Candy pointed toward the cluster of dogwoods and hickory trees just beyond her patio. "In the spring those dogwoods are just filled with blooms—and everything is covered with a yellow pollen from the hickory trees. So I knew my problem must be allergy related. I kept going to doctor after doctor. Finally, the year before I was diagnosed with cancer, I had surgery on my sinuses.

"I knew something wasn't right when, after I had recovered from the surgery, the pain was worse than ever. My sinuses had been drained, and X rays the doctors took showed that they were clear. But the pain got worse. Not only that, my worst sinus had been the left one, and now most of the pain was on the right side."

It was at this point that Candy first began to wonder if her pain could be caused by a tumor. "It just didn't feel like a sinus headache. I had been having sinus headaches for fifteen years. This felt like something different. But I was told that usually only seventy-year-olds get tumors in their sinuses."

Nevertheless the pain persisted, accompanied by several intense nosebleeds. "They were gushers!" Candy exclaimed. "I had to go to the emergency room three times for nosebleeds." Physically active, she had taught and practiced dance for years. Nevertheless, she began losing weight. "I thought, *That's not good for me.* I was down to ninety-two pounds."

At this point, even though Candy wasn't aware that she had cancer, she began experiencing one of the emotions experienced most by cancer patients—anxiety. One of the most common human emotions, anxiety has a lot in common with fear. As Dr. Koppersmith frequently tells the patients in his psychiatric practice, "Both anxiety and fear are emotions that relate to uncertainties about the future. The difference is, fear usually has a specific object—something like cancer. On the other hand, when we are anxious, we are often unaware of just what it is that triggers our concern."

Anxiety: A Distracting Concern

The biblical concept of anxiety is of a distracting concern. The actual word employed by Jesus and the writers of the New Testament to describe anxiety and warn against it comes from a verb meaning to "have a distracting care."[1] Distraction is precisely what Candy Wood began to experience.

"It got to be such a hassle—running from doctor to doctor. I was happily married, enjoyed my two children—but I just couldn't shake this physical problem or get rid of the pain. And I kept thinking, *What could be wrong with me?* You know, going over and over the question in my mind."

After living with her pain and anxiety for months, Candy was finally told by her physician that she had a "pea-sized" growth in her nasal cavity. "I thought, *Hot dog! We found it. This is it—this is why I hurt.*" Deciding to try to deal with the pain for another month before undergoing surgery so that she and her husband could take a planned vacation, Candy found her anxiety level increasing. "I hadn't even thought of cancer, because you just don't think of cancer in the head. No one in my family had cancer. Or even my friends. But I was concerned. Underneath I knew something wasn't right—the anxiety just kept nagging at me."

Finally, in the spring of 1982, Candy's anxiety became real fear. She had just returned to Birmingham from the ski trip to Colorado. "It was a hot, muggy day—extremely humid. I was miserable. My head was killing me, and I thought, *I'm going to another stupid doctor's office.*" The pain was still there, greater than ever, permeating her head.

Convinced that her problem had to be something more than allergies, Candy remembers that first visit to Dr. Poyner like it was yesterday. "I felt so irritated sitting in his office. The waiting room was sort of a sixties tacky-orange and chartreuse leather, and contemporary chairs with steel arms. The floor was a creamy gray tile. Not at all the plush office common today."

After what seemed an extremely long wait, Candy was finally invited to step into the examining room. "I thought, *It's freezing in here. No wonder he has patients—he's giving them pneumonia.*" Then the doctor walked in, slim, midforties, obviously a gentleman, wearing tortoise-shell glasses, a bow tie, and a red lab coat. "I remember thinking, *Why is he wearing that red lab coat? I guess he must see a lot of children.*"

Anger and Denial: A Normal Response

Candy was shocked at what he said after the examination. "I want you in the hospital yesterday."

"What? What do you mean, you want me in the hospital yesterday?" At which point, Candy, a self-described Southern lady, reacted in what she termed very unladylike fashion. She looked him in the eye and told him, "All you doctors want to do is operate."

"OK, I'll call my partner in."

In a few minutes, Dr. Poyner returned with his partner, Dr. Goldfarb. "He was a really handsome Jewish man—tanned, dark eyes, kind face, wearing a royal-blue lab jacket and a paisley tie," Candy noted.

Although his appearance was strikingly different from Dr. Poyner's, Dr. Goldfarb voiced the same opinion as his colleague. After he examined Candy he said, "You need to be in the hospital right now."

Suddenly, for the first time, the dreaded word crept into Candy's vocabulary. "It can't be cancer or anything, can it?" By her own admission, Candy's remark was asked in a way designed to draw a negative response. "But all they said was, 'We don't think so, but that's why we want to do a biopsy.'

"I was so . . . so mad."

Dr. Poyner asked, "When would you like us to schedule your surgery for the biopsy, Candy?"

"I don't. I can't. I don't have time. I have other things to do—a dance recital for my students, tons of things to finish up before the end of the school year."

Both physicians were insistent. "We want you in. When do you want us to schedule it?"

Equally adamant, Candy replied, "I'm not going anywhere."

After this intense verbal exchange, Dr. Poyner ushered Candy from the examination room to his office. She noticed that his desk was neatly stacked with papers and books. Paintings covered the walls. "He was an avid art collector," she remembered.

As soon as they were seated, Dr. Poyner asked, "What's your husband's telephone number?"

Candy couldn't believe what happened next. "Lee, my husband, was home with the flu. There I was, in this doctor's office. He's sitting there across the desk from me, on the phone, telling my husband I need to be in surgery tomorrow. I thought, *I'm not doing this. Who does he think he is, telling my husband that I'm going to surgery? I haven't agreed to any surgery at all!*"

Candy responded to her anger with an all-too-common defense—denial.

Candy remembers her intense feeling of anger. "When I left his office I didn't say, 'Thank you for your time. Thank you for your concern.' Nothing. And that's just not like me. I remember slamming the door as I walked out of the doctor's office, then slamming the car door."

As she was to learn later, Candy's anger was a normal response. Anger is the emotion we feel in response to a threat —a threat to our lives, our well-being, our loved ones, even our significance. In this case, Candy was confronted with an unthinkable threat. Prior to that springtime visit to Dr. Poyner's office, the words *cancer* and *biopsy* hadn't even been part of her working vocabulary. Suddenly, all the rules were changed. She was threatened, and she responded with anger.

But like many cancer victims, including a high proportion of Christians, Candy responded to her anger with an all-too-common defense—denial. "I went home to Lee—he was in bed sick with the flu. And he says, 'What's the deal, this doctor telling you you need to have surgery?'

"I said, 'Forget it. If you don't want me to have it, I won't have it. Right now I need to be at the studio.'" Making every effort to put the whole affair out of her mind, Candy packed up her things and drove off to the Steeple Arts Studio where she taught dance.

Denial is one of the most dangerous responses for the cancer patient. It comes in many shapes and sizes—all dangerous. It can insert itself into just about any point in the process, from diagnosis to treatment. Denial can keep a person just diagnosed with cancer from seeking a second opinion, or even agreeing to treatment. It has caused many a suspected cancer patient to reject even having a biopsy.

When a patient has been told that he or she might have cancer, intense emotions are an expected response—anger at the diagnosis, anxiety about the future, a sense of loneliness, of isolation from others who are healthy, and, beneath it all, an intense, overwhelming fear. After all, fear is commonly considered by psychiatrists and psychologists to be the basic emotion that underlies most others, such as anger. Fear is the very first emotion identified in the Bible, an emotion closely associated with the aftereffects of mankind's fall into sin.

Picture the scene in the Garden of Eden: Adam and Eve, crouching in the underbrush, trying to hide from God, whose voice lovingly frames the question to which He already knows the answer: "Adam, where are you?"

"Lord, I decided we should hide, since we were unclothed. After all, I was afraid."

There it is, almost as an aside: the first admission of a negative emotion—fear. Fear of the consequences of their nakedness. At a more basic level, fear of God and of the result of their disobedience. He had, after all, warned them: "In the day you eat the forbidden fruit, you will die." Ever since that early point in human history, men and women have been fearing death . . . and pain and rejection and failure and a host of other things, not the least of which is cancer.

Denial is a false refuge,
a dead-end street.
Denial can kill.

Dr. Wendy Schelessel Harpham, an internist who practices in Dallas, felt happy in her work, fulfilled in her home life, and in excellent health. Then one day she developed intense pain in her groin and back. The diagnosis? Disseminated lymphoma, cancer that had originated in the lymph nodes and spread throughout her body.

Dr. Harpham candidly described her initial emotions as "Numbing shock, primal fear, and childlike helplessness." As she later admitted, "Graphic memories of past patients deprived me of the strength and comfort that came from denial." She explained: "A major reason why denial is such a common emotional response in cancer patients is that it seems to provide the only strength and comfort. That's why it's so common for patients who have been told they have cancer and must receive treatment to retreat into what they perceive to be the safe shelter of denial."[2] But denial is a false refuge, a dead-end street. Denial can kill.

For instance, a man named Ellis refused to admit that there was any possibility he could have cancer. Sure, he had been more tired than usual and had passed blood in his stool on quite a few occasions. Hemorrhoids, that's what he attributed his problem to.

Refusing his physician's recommendation of sigmoidoscopy, a procedure to examine the colon and lower bowel, or even a simple routine hemoccult check for signs of colorectal cancer, Ellis retreated into what he thought was the comfort of denial. Two years later, he lost his battle with cancer. Prolonged denial had tipped the scales against him—and many others like him.

Into the Hospital

Candy chose not to remain in denial, at least not for long. "I kept flip-flopping back and forth between anger and denial. The day I went in for surgery I told my husband, 'Don't worry. It's just a one-day thing. I'm going on over to St. Vincent's Hospital this morning. You come on over after work. It's no big deal, really.'" There Candy was, trying to convince everybody that it was no big deal. But deep inside, things were different. "I was nervous. Really scared."

Candy was due at the hospital at 3:00 P.M. That morning, she and her two-year-old daughter Colley took a bike ride down the scenic road that led from their home toward Crestline Village. The skies over Birmingham had turned dark, threatening a thunderstorm. "But I decided to go ahead, riding my bike. I wanted to have the time with Colley. And I had other plans. I planned to run by the Crestline Elementary School and kiss

Elliott, my son, good-bye before I went to the hospital. He was going to a birthday party. And my sister-in-law had just had a baby the night before, so I needed to stop by and see her at Montclair Hospital. That was the plan."

But as Candy and her daughter rode the bike down the hill into Crestline Village, the owner of one of the stores flagged her down to tell her that her mother was looking for her and had phoned his store. "So I called Mother back. She told me St. Vincent's Hospital had just called. They wanted me to come in earlier—for tests. So I thought, *Whoa! They want me to have tests? Who? And why? What's the deal here. I don't want to go for tests, and I'm just not gonna do it. I'm sticking with the original plan. I'll go see Elliott, then visit my sister-in-law at the other hospital. Then I'll go to St. Vincent's.*"

Looking back on that day, Candy cataloged her emotions at that point. "By now, I was really upset—belligerent, fired up, and scared. All the above."

Candy remembered finally arriving at the entrance to St. Vincent's Hospital an hour after the time they had requested. It was pouring rain—the impending thunderstorm had broken just as Candy's mother dropped her off—at Candy's insistence —at the entrance to the hospital. Candy kissed her mother and Colley good-bye, then watched her mother drive off into the pouring rain. Her conscious thoughts were *This is no big deal.* But inside she felt so frightened, so alone.

The May thunderstorm that had obliterated the Birmingham skyline was nothing compared to the storm of emotion that was about to break loose inside Candy. She entered the hospital, completed her paperwork, then was placed on a machine for tomography—a series of three-dimensional photographs that provide physicians with much better diagnostic information than used to be available—information that could previously be obtained only by exploratory surgery.

The storm of emotion first struck as Candy observed the response of the technician who carried out the tomography. "It takes a while, you know—all those click-click-clicks. Well, that left me pretty scared. Then I thought, *The guy must be seeing something.* He kept taking even more pictures. So I asked him, 'What do you see? Do you see something?' I just knew he had seen something. But all he would tell me is, 'A radiologist can tell you. I'm not supposed to say anything.' That was enough to really freak me out—*I just know he's definitely seeing something, but he won't tell me. He just says, 'We're not allowed to say anything.'*"

A short time later, as she waited in her room in a new wing of the hospital, Dr. Goldfarb walked through the door. Candy remembers his words vividly: "It looks like from the tomography and the other tests that we're dealing with something bigger than just a cyst. It looks like it's more the size of a golf ball. It's invaded the whole sinus cavity."

Still in denial, Candy's response was, "So? You just take out a bigger cyst, right? No problem."

"The real issue of my fear was that I equated cancer with death."

Dr. Goldfarb's response was so measured and careful that Candy said, "OK, give me the bottom line. What's the worst thing that can happen to me?"

Looking her squarely in the eye, Dr. Goldfarb replied, "You could lose the right side of your face."

"Why? It can't be cancer, can it?" Candy was thinking all the while that he'd say, "That's right, it can't be."

Again, Dr. Goldfarb paused and looked at Candy. "Yes, it definitely *can* be cancer. But you asked for the worst, so let's just hope for the best."

"The moment Dr. Goldfarb walked out the door I went into a major panic attack. I began calling everybody—my parents, pastor, other doctors—I just wanted somebody to fix this—right now."

Suddenly, ominously, terrifyingly, Candy's fear had taken shape. "And it wasn't the fear of losing my face—even though looks had always been an important thing with me. The real issue of my fear was that I equated cancer with death."

Following an intense outburst of emotion, a feverish conversation with her husband, impassioned pleas by telephone to physicians, family, pastors, and friends, Candy was finally given a sleeping pill, which allowed her temporary respite from the storm of emotion.

Emotional Roller Coaster

Candy and Liz (story in chapter 2) both identified one more emotion that is extremely common for cancer patients—depression. The phrase both used to explain their feelings were almost identical—"It's like being on an emotional roller coaster." That's the phrase Liz used to describe how she felt as she sat in her oncologist's office during a follow-up visit after successful surgery for lung cancer. Candy used the same words that fall afternoon as she thought back over the seven years of treatment for the malignant mass the doctors had removed from behind her right eye.

Sitting in her den that gloomy fall afternoon describing her seven-year ordeal, Candy talked about intense highs and lows. "I think the reason I started on the roller coaster was that I'm sort of an all-or-nothing person. I'm either totally involved in a project or I don't get involved at all. No middle of the road for me.

"In fact, I have several friends who have some kind of handicap or other. I used to tell them if I were ever handicapped I'd be the best handicapped person in the world—totally involved. Or I would just go into a room somewhere, watch TV, and vegetate.

"So when this cancer thing first hit me, I decided if I was to be a cancer patient, and maybe be disfigured and have to go to the Mayo Clinic, I was gonna be the most positive, the most go-for-it cancer patient there ever was. That was my attitude from day two in the hospital. I went from being very upset to very up. But then Wednesday stretched into Thursday—and definite results still hadn't come back from the biopsy." Candy was experiencing an incredible combination of stresses. Her life had been disrupted. All the plans for working with her dance students, spending time with her family, getting on with her life were now on hold.

In addition, it seemed to Candy that no one fully understood what was wrong. Numerous medical doctors just hadn't been able to figure out her problem. That left Candy even more uncertain about herself, her condition, and her future. "At the time I couldn't imagine what I was about to go through for the next seven years. My personality is such that you give me one little ray of hope and I'll hang on to it every time. But I lay there in that bed all that Thursday, after the biopsy surgery. At first I wanted to figure this out—see how I could fix this problem. But then I kept thinking, over and over, *I've been seeing all those doctors. How could they all have missed this?* Nothing was computing. I couldn't seem to get to the bottom of it. *How did it happen?*"

Then, as she struggled with the stresses and losses the situation had caused, her inability to understand what was wrong, and the uncertainty about when and how she would get better, Candy experienced another of the factors that leaves so many cancer patients depressed—a frightening and painful experience during the course of treatment. All that Thursday Candy had tried to figure out her situation. So by 9:30 that evening, she was both physically and mentally exhausted. Listen as she describes what happened next.

"At this point, the third partner in Dr. Poyner's ENT group, Dr. Gerwin, came in to pull out the packing from my nose. I expected him to remove a little gauze pad—you know, something small. Instead, he ripped out over seventy inches of gauze from my nose. And that did it! He just kept ripping and ripping, and I started crying hysterically." The combination of the physical pain and discomfort, coupled with the emotional implications, had plunged Candy to the depths of despair.

"I kept on crying hysterically—and by one or two o'clock, in the middle of the night, I felt like I'd had it. I mean, that was just the end of Candy, totally—emotionally, spiritually, mentally, physically. My face was swollen, and on top of that the nurses had lost my chart. They didn't know what they could give me and couldn't find a doctor to ask. They weren't aware that they could pack my face with ice to keep it from swelling."

Ironically, Candy pointed to the depth of her depression as the crisis point where things began to turn for the better. "After all, I'd always been pretty good at manipulating things— trying to figure them out, then figuring out how to fix them. It was at the point of my deepest despair that I just totally gave in to the Lord. I told Him, 'Lord, I don't care what You do—You accomplish whatever You want with me. You make the decisions. I'm sure not capable of making them.'" So in the wee hours of that morning, lying in a hospital bed with occasional muted sounds of people in the hallway, the whispered feet of nurses, the quiet hum of air conditioning equipment, Candy, at her point of ultimate despair, turned things over to the Lord.

All that night, Candy had been alone, except for her mother who was sitting up with her. After hours of tears and crying, pleas and despair, Candy's mother had stepped out to grab a quick cup of coffee. Candy seemed asleep. When her mother quietly slipped back into the room, Candy looked up and in a calm voice said, "Mama, I don't know where this came from, other than the Lord. But all I can tell you is, what I'm about to go through is going to be so horrible people won't believe it. But it will be OK in the end." Describing the moment later, Candy added, "And I knew it! I knew it was true."

A popular working definition of depression [is] "emotions, such as anger, turned inward."

Candy would look back on this as the key turning point in dealing with her emotions. There would still be times of anger, periods of depression, bouts with anxiety and fear. "But that was the time when I told my mother I knew I would make it. It would be terrible, but I would be OK in the end. Now I'm not a great theologian, haven't been to seminary. But I believed God had given me peace, and, if I felt such assurance, it had to have come supernaturally from the Lord."

Candy's experience fits remarkably with Paul's promise of emotional peace and stability found in Philippians 4. As he encourages his readers to stop being anxious, Paul calls on them to express their concerns and requests to God in a prayerful, thankful manner (v. 6). Then he promises them God's remarkable peace, which is beyond human understanding, to serve as a guardian of their emotions and thought processes (v. 7).

During those early morning hours, Candy came to the end of her anxieties, her efforts, her fears. Knowing she had no other workable alternative, she turned them over to God. And at that point, God's peace began to guard and sustain her emotions and her mind.

To the Mayo Clinic

That didn't mean Candy would never again experience an emotional roller coaster. In a matter of days she would find herself on a plane bound from Birmingham to the Mayo Clinic in Rochester, Minnesota, where she would be whisked into one of the fifty-three operating rooms at nearby St. Mary's Hospital, surrounded by nurses and technicians in stark white uniforms, white stockings, and white shoes.

Dr. Ian Jackson, an internationally respected surgeon from Scotland, would perform an incredible surgical procedure, removing her entire face with the exception of her mouth and two eyes, leaving Candy severely deformed. That surgery took more than nine hours. Dr. Jackson excised a malignant mass the size of a baseball from behind her right eye, plus all her nearby facial bones. Those bones were rushed to the lab, where they were checked for malignancy. When they were found to be cancer free, Dr. Jackson, who specializes in reconstructive surgery on children, decided to reconstruct the right side of Candy's face.

Candy and her husband, Lee, were both amazed by her appearance following the surgery. Stitches ran across her face from ear to ear; another row of sutures curved around her nose. But she still had her face. Back home, during the recuperative process, Candy's emotional roller-coaster ride continued. "One minute I'd be all fired up—full of faith and hope. The next I'd be exhausted, frightened, discouraged, and teary."

An additional factor in Candy's emotional roller coaster was the belief that she needed to perform for others in order to maintain a good testimony, despite intense, recurring facial pain, which was a sign of impending infection. "I so wanted God to bring good things out of what I had been through. I thought I needed to help Him do that, so I pretty much limited my complaining to my husband."

Most clinical professionals employ a popular working definition of depression as "emotions, such as anger, turned inward." Both Candy and Lee experienced a significant degree of depression, a normal response to such traumatic events. Candy's limited energy resources as she recuperated from the surgery, plus the increasing pain, made it difficult to cope. Even though she was a people person and enjoyed having numerous family members and friends around the house to help with children, meals, and cleaning, neither Candy nor Lee could get much rest. Lee found himself angry—angry at the disruption in the household, angry at Candy because of her illness, even angry at God. Although it was difficult for her to admit, Candy was experiencing some of the same emotions—plus struggling inside with guilt over feeling those emotions.

Compounded Emotions

We have found this "compounding" of emotions to be one of the most significant components in the emotional impact of cancer. It is extremely common in conscientious Christians who feel they must joyfully accept whatever circumstances come their way, yet who struggle with grief over the loss of health, appearance, and personal freedoms, and anger at physicians, family members, and God.

---

*"Cancer surgery is not like
an appendectomy, where you go in,
have the surgery, go home and get well,
and that's it."*

Ironically, both Candy and Lee began to work through their depression during the time when Candy was forced to return to the Mayo Clinic to undergo four additional surgeries over a thirty-five day period—surgeries performed to remove infected material and graft skin from Candy's thighs over the back and side of her head. "It was an incredibly difficult five weeks. But during that time I grew closer to the Lord than I ever had been. I think one of the keys was thankfulness—I kept remembering that I still had my face, and could still see through both my eyes. I was lifted by my prayers, and by those of my family and friends."

For both Candy and Lee there would still be times of discouragement and depression—even outbursts of anger, times of pain and fatigue, and struggles with the fear of a recurrence of the cancer that dealt such a devastating blow to Candy and Lee's lives. "It was like a black cloud, continuing to hang over us. I don't know about all the other cancer patients, but cancer surgery is not like an appendectomy, where you go in, have the surgery, go home and get well, and that's it. With cancer, you go in, and even *if* they get it, you still may need more treatment —you know, drag it out. Then every three months or every six months or whatever intervals your doctors say, you have to go back, and they look for more cancer."

For Candy, the checkups came at three-month intervals. For two-and-a-half months, she was able to maintain a cheerful stability to handle her anxiety, fear, and depression. "Then two weeks before time for the trip back to Mayo, you could see my personality change, even though I would say, 'God's in control. I have faith.' I would immerse myself in studying the Scriptures and have people praying, but there still was that underlying fear. The recognition that I was going back so they could look for it again. So there's the possibility they may find it."

Candy didn't revert back to her original denial—not back to "I don't have cancer, do I?" but back to the emotional thunderstorm that so resembled the physical storm that broke over St. Vincent's Hospital on the Birmingham skyline the day she first underwent surgery for her massive tumor. "It's just always like a big, black storm cloud. Something hanging over you."

Coping with Emotions

The emotional component of cancer provides one of the greatest challenges to the cancer patient—and the patient's family and friends. Although the physical effects of cancer are generally recognized, frequently the emotional component is overlooked. For that reason, we recommend the following steps to deal with the emotional implications of cancer.

1 *Break through any lingering denial.* Whenever we are confronted with any unpleasant truth, our normal response is denial. Found at the top of the classic list of defense mechanisms,[3] *denial* is defined as a mechanism in which the existence of unpleasant realities is disavowed. The term refers to a keeping out of conscious awareness any aspects of external reality that, if acknowledged, would produce anxiety.

Denial is at the root of the entire human dilemma, since it involves the inner person's ability to exercise self-deceit regarding threatening negative elements in our environment. Many centuries ago the prophet Jeremiah linked this capacity for self-deception to the human sin nature (Jeremiah 17:9). In confronting his harshest critics—the Pharisees—Jesus Christ pinpointed their denial of their own serious spiritual deficiencies as the prime factor in their spiritual bondage, pointing out to them that acknowledging the truth would set them free (John 8:32). Unfortunately, they chose to continue denying the very need with which they were confronted. The apostle John, who recorded this confrontation between Christ and the religious leaders of His day over the issue of denial, identifies this defense in his first epistle as a serious problem—and an ongoing risk—for Christians (1 John 1:8, 10).

Though Scripture addresses denial from a spiritual perspective, this defense can have harmful implications for the cancer patient as well. We have already cataloged how Candy Wood struggled with denial and how it took extraordinary circumstances for her to face the serious reality of her condition. Unfortunately, Candy's response is not unusual—denial is incredibly common and extremely dangerous. As we have already noted, denial, when mixed with cancer, can kill, since time is often of the essence in dealing with malignancy. If there is any possibility that you have cancer, or if you have been told that you do, it is extremely important to face the truth, no matter how unpleasant or frightening. Ironically, the truth is often not as bad as we anticipate it to be. Yet even if this is not the case, we cannot really move toward dealing with the emotional, or even the physical, components of our cancer until we break through the denial barrier.

2 *Share feelings honestly with those who are close to you.* We live in a society that magnifies self-reliance, even idealizes in some ways the Lone Ranger approach to dealing with problems. Yet even the Lone Ranger relied on his faithful companion, Tonto, and his trusted horse, Silver. They were as important to him as his Colt revolver that he loaded with silver bullets.

We have found that so many cancer patients feel like the Lone Ranger, or worse. All too often the numbness of denial is replaced by the gnawing ache of isolation, the intense feeling that no one else fully knows, understands, or cares. For Candy, sharing the burden with her husband, her mother, and special friends from her church family provided crucial support to deal with the ongoing battle.

Solomon speaks of a friend who "loves at all times" and that a brother is born for adversity (Proverbs 17:17). Proverbs 27 is filled with wise sayings about friendship, sayings that hold particular significance for the cancer patient. Friends who are loyal (v. 10), who provide encouraging delight (v. 9), who are honest enough to lovingly tell the truth even when it is painful (v. 6), who recognize when it is time to back off (v. 14), and who ultimately are part of the sharpening and strengthening process (v. 17) provide an incredible resource for those who struggle with cancer. If you have been diagnosed with cancer, closely examine these statements from Proverbs—perhaps in a modern translation. Then look for friends and family members who can help meet these support needs in your life.

This is not to minimize the role of Scripture, prayer, or the support provided by the Holy Spirit who indwells every believer. God has provided these resources as our first line of defense for whatever comes our way, as well as keys to spiritual and personal growth. Yet the many "one another" passages in Scripture make clear that we are also to be dependent on others, particularly those of "like precious faith" (2 Peter 1:1).

3 *Spread the sharing of your burdens around.* Emotional overload is one of the major hazards we have noticed for those who are close to cancer patients. This often leads to roller-coaster emotions. One of the things we discovered when talking with Candy Wood about her cancer was the burden she placed on her husband. As she put it, "I felt free to complain to Lee. With everyone else, I just performed. He didn't get a lot of rest, nor did he have anyone to talk to about his own feelings."

As Candy unloaded more and more of her emotional burden on Lee, and as he struggled under the weight of having little or no emotional support, things finally came to a head in an explosive incident that left Lee enraged and Candy in tears. By spreading the burden around, not overloading one or two primary resources, the cancer patient can help assure more effective long-term and encouraging support from those primary significant others.

4 *Seek out a support group.* Cancer recovery support groups can now be found in just about every part of the country. In many cases, local churches and other organizations provide a Christian perspective for encouragement and support. The morning after their blow-up, Candy's husband called to obtain information about a support group. Both learned important lessons from participating in the group. Candy came to understand that Lee needed her time and attention. Lee learned how to deal with his fears, questions, and anger, rather than simply bottling his emotions up until they boiled over. And both learned, as Candy put it, to "communicate our own needs to each other and be sensitive to each other's needs."

5 *Seek counseling.* For many individuals the grief associated with the diagnosis of cancer, plus related physical and emotional stresses, peels away the scars from deep-seated emotional wounds of the past. For such individuals, the insight and wisdom of a counselor is extremely helpful. Since Proverbs teaches that only the wise seek counsel (Proverbs 12:15), there should be no stigma attached to seeking out counsel. We have recommended professional or pastoral counseling to literally hundreds of people who have been diagnosed with cancer and to their families with good results. We've also experienced its benefits firsthand.

6 *Plan on recurrences of emotional ups-and-downs.* Candy Wood made it clear that during the ordeal of her multiple surgeries, and for years afterward, there was a continuing emotional roller-coaster experience. Whenever she faced her three-month checkup, she would sense those negative emotions building. A cancer patient needs to plan to have adequate support to continue dealing with the emotional stress and trauma, even after being declared cancer free.

7 *Check for physical components of depression.* Certain forms of cancer, such as the pancreatic variety experienced by Cliff (chapter 3) and Doc (story in chapter 9), can actually trigger a clinical depression. It's important to discuss this with an oncologist and, if necessary, be referred to a psychiatrist for appropriate medical treatment.

8 *Regain hope.* Remember that cancer is not a death sentence. Candy Wood discovered this truth for herself. "I realized that I wasn't doomed to die—that there was hope for survival and

even a positive quality of life. That made all the difference in the world."

Scripture is filled with evidences of the hope we have in Jesus Christ and with principles for applying this hope to our lives. Three times during the darkest time of his personal difficulties, David reminded himself, "Hope in God, for I shall yet praise Him for the help of His countenance" (Psalm 42:5; 42:11; 43:5). In Lamentations 3:21–25, Jeremiah regains emotional and spiritual perspective in the middle of a grave personal and national disaster by refocusing from *his* circumstances to *God's* loyal love and tender compassions. "The Lord is my portion," he said, "therefore I hope in Him" (v. 24).

Whereas those who are not Christians can develop a measure of hope, only those who genuinely know Christ can experience the living hope to which we have been reborn—a hope based on the indisputable fact of the resurrection of Christ. Such hope can sustain us through a variety of personal trials and adversities (1 Peter 1:3, 6) and actually give us cause for rejoicing in adversity since we know that God's purpose is not to disappoint us but to lovingly develop us (Romans 5:2–5). It was Candy Wood's steadfast hope, based on her faith in Jesus Christ, that sustained her during the dark days when she feared death from the cancer that had invaded her body. Then her hope motivated her to reach out to encourage others not to give in to their disfigurement or the debilitating effects of the disease.

9 *Keep processing your feelings.* In talking with those who have a great deal of emotional trauma to process, we frequently encounter the question, "Why can't I just do something once and for all to deal with all this emotional baggage? Why can't God just zap me and get rid of everything?" We gently remind them that the problem is *not* God's inability to deal with things once and for all. However, His loving purpose is usually to take us through the process. Part of that process involves dealing biblically with anger and other feelings.

Paul's reminder in Ephesians 4 about how to deal with anger appropriately has tremendous implications for the cancer patient. After warning against the danger of denial and other forms of deceit (v. 25), Paul encourages his readers in Ephesus to "be angry, and do not sin: do not let the sun go down on your wrath, nor give place to the devil" (vv. 26–27). Frequently the grudges we harbor toward those around us, toward ourselves or even toward God, can cause ongoing emotional trauma, intensified physical difficulties, and significant spiritual deterioration as Satan gains a foothold in our lives.

The alternative we recommend is to daily become aware of the anger we have within, just as Paul warned us, and to process that anger in a timely fashion. We sometimes use the illustration of peeling an onion to help make this process clear. When a housewife peels an onion, she may pull back the visible, outer layer, only to discover another layer underneath— and still another layer beneath that one. Peeling an onion is frequently accompanied by tears, and, if there are scratches on the hands, by intense pain. Furthermore, the process can seem endless, as layer after layer is brought to light, then peeled away. Ultimately however, as the process is continued, the final layer is exposed, the core of the onion is reached, and the task is completed. Emotionally, we consider this the point at which healing has occurred. The scars are still present, but the intense emotions we call "resentment," or "re-feeling" of the initial emotions, no longer occur. We encourage cancer patients to continue processing their emotions with this goal in mind.

10 *Work toward acceptance and peace.* One of the most difficult emotional components for the cancer patient is to come to grips with the reality that cancer, one way or another, will be a part of his or her life from now on. In that sense, the cancer diagnosis becomes a personal watershed. Frequently the patient has great difficulty coming to terms with this.

In his excellent article on the cancer experience and stages of grief, Donald Nichols, academic dean of the Oakland Community College in Farmington Hills, Michigan, writes about the final stage of grief, which is acceptance, providing a combination of personal experience and clinical perspective: "All of my contacts reported great relief on moving on to this last stage. The magnified emotional response which dominated previous stages was lifted, and a sense of ease was attained. No longer was the affective domain dominant in their experiences, as they were now able to intellectually deal with their circumstances."[4]

We identify what Nichols is talking about as coming to peace with the reality of your cancer. From a spiritual perspective, this is the goal of Christians in every area of adversity. According to the apostle Paul, it is secured by continuing to turn from anxiety to prayer (Philippians 4:6–7). Certainly the intense anxiety, the ongoing stress, the strong anger, and other emotions that are by-products of cancer must be dealt with appropriately. (We will have more to say on the subject of the spiritual component in the next chapter.)

The obvious joy on the face of Candy Wood—a face that still bore the scars of massive craniofacial surgery, weeks of bone infection, and additional operations to deal with the recurring infection—spoke clearly of her success in dealing with the emotional trauma of cancer. Candy did not focus on the looks she had lost, but rather on what she had left. She possessed life and energy, plus skills and techniques she had learned from her theatre days in college, that enabled her to develop make-up techniques to help minimize her disfigurement. And by processing her emotions appropriately, Candy had peace.

Candy's peace is not a passive fatalism but rather an active go-for-it approach to life that involves making the most of her situation, reaching out to help and encourage others, and recognizing that God does in fact have a positive purpose, despite the incredible negative aspects of her experience with cancer. In short, Candy has come to terms—to peace—with her cancer experience.

7

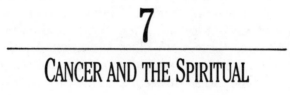 CANCER AND THE SPIRITUAL

Liz was sitting up in bed, a tray of bland-looking hospital food in front of her, when Karla tiptoed into the room in response to a muffled "Come on in." Several potted plants and floral arrangements gave the room the appearance of a botanical garden. One entire wall was covered with crudely fashioned children's drawings, along with a variety of cards produced by Hallmark and Dayspring.

Across the room from the bed, a television newscaster soundlessly described the day's significant events. Occasional images of starving African children and military vehicles periodically replaced his features. Although the window curtains were pulled shut, shafts of brilliant sunshine thrust their way into the dimly lit room.

"Thanks for coming, Karla," Liz said as she pushed her tray back. "You timed it perfectly—I just finished. I'm still not able to hold much food. But you know how they treat you after surgery these days. Get you up and walking right away. Try to start you on foods so they can get rid of the IV."

"Not like when *I* had surgery," Karla replied. Tall and willowy, with a few natural streaks of gray in her curly brown hair, Karla walked across the room and placed an envelope with the name *Liz* written calligraphy-style on the front. "Now don't open this until after I leave."

"Well, let's not talk about your leaving, girl. After all, you just got here. And I haven't seen a soul besides Bill and the doctors—well, other than my sister and her husband."

A grimace darkened Liz's face as she remembered the visit the previous evening. "Actually, I'm glad you're here, Karla. I have a lot of respect for you. I mean, you're the one who got me started in that Bible study class at church. And I've always admired your attitude, even when you had cancer. It just didn't seem to shake you. So sit down and let me pick your brain for a while."

Smiling, Karla moved to the olive-colored fabric chair Liz indicated, pulled it closer to the bed, and seated herself. "I'm not sure I'd agree that I handled my cancer all that well, Liz. But I sure am a lot farther down the road now. So tell me about what's weighing on your mind."

Liz paused a moment to take a sip from the water glass on the nearby food tray, then pressed the button that elevated her higher in the hospital bed. She took a deep breath and began her explanation. "Bill and I are Christians, you know. We've tried to serve God with our family and our work. We haven't been perfect, but . . ." Her voice broke, and Liz dabbed a tear from the edge of her left eye. After a moment she blurted out, "Do you really think this cancer is God's way of judging me for some sin in my life? Or if I had enough faith, God would heal me immediately?"

Karla frowned as Liz continued her questions. "Do you think there may be something in my life I don't even know about that's made God angry at me?"

After a moment, Liz began to sob gently. Karla reached over and took her hand but didn't say anything. Before long, Liz regained her composure, but her voice was still taut with emotion. "Go ahead, Karla. Feel free to tell me what a sinner I am. Maybe God's just mad at me because I kept asking Him why."

Karla resisted the temptation to respond to her hurting friend with a pious platitude. Instead, she waited for a moment, then gently said, "Tell me about it, Liz. Maybe I can help most by just listening."

Tears flowed again for a moment. Then Liz regained her composure. "Sorry, Karla. I didn't intend for things to come out like that. I really shouldn't dump this on you."

"Hold on Liz," Karla replied firmly. "Who said anything about dumping? I'm your friend, right?"

Liz nodded.

"And didn't *I* share things with *you* when we lost Suzie in that accident last year?"

Remembering the pain of her friend's grief, Liz smiled weakly, nodding as she grasped her friend's hand. "We went through it together, didn't we?"

"We sure did," Karla continued. "And I want to go through this with you. After all, that's what friends are for—especially Christian friends. So why don't you tell me about this feeling you have that God is mad at you or that your cancer is the result of some terrible sin you've committed or a lack of faith."

"Well, I've sort of had these nagging thoughts in the back of my mind ever since Dr. Franklin first told me about the possibility of cancer. Then, when Bill and I talked to Dr. Morris, they became even more intense. So I asked Bill if he thought God could be punishing me for something. But he told me he didn't think so. Of course, he doesn't talk a lot about spiritual things, you know. I'm convinced he's a man of strong faith. And I know he loves me. He's like a lot of men—sort of a man of few words."

Karla nodded, smiling. "That's the way Jake is too. I thought he'd never be able to talk about it when we lost Suzie—or even cry. But he finally did. But if Bill didn't give you this idea about God's judgment, who did?"

Liz hesitated a moment, taking another sip of water. "I guess my sister and her husband started me thinking about it. They came by last night. Didn't stay long. And they didn't exactly accuse me of hiding some sin. It's sort of what they implied, more than what they said."

"What do you mean?" Karla asked, a puzzled look on her face.

"Well, you'd have to know my sister and her husband. I mean, they're really strong Christians, I'm sure. I've always respected them for their faith and their zeal. They're so involved in their church. But it's like they're just absolutely convinced that it's always God's will to heal anybody who's sick. They told me one of God's names was Jehovah Rapha, and that means *the Lord who heals*. They even read some verses to me—from

Exodus. They said something like, 'He would heal us from all diseases, because He is Jehovah Rapha.' They didn't come out and say this about me, but a couple of times during the conversation they both hinted that the only reason Christians weren't healed from their sickness was because they didn't have enough faith or they had some hidden sin."

Liz brushed her hair back from her face. "Karla, I just don't know what to think. If there's some hidden sin in my life, I want to deal with it. I don't want anything to come between me and God. The doctor suggested that I have a long fight against cancer ahead of me. So help me figure this out."

Pulling a small, maroon Bible from one of the pockets in her large brown handbag, Karla snapped it open and began turning pages until she reached the book of Exodus. She looked up when Liz, grinning, said, "You always come prepared, don't you?"

Karla nodded. "Here's the part that talks about Jehovah Rapha. Do you want to look at it, or would you rather I read it to you?"

"Just read it to me—and help me figure out what it means for me," Liz said tiredly.

"Interpretation and application?"

"After we observe the text," Liz smiled, perking up.

"Well, you remember the first thing we have to do is look at the context. Let's see, Exodus 14:22 suggests that Israel has just come out of Egypt through the Red Sea. They went into the wilderness and couldn't find any water. Then they found some bitter water at a place called Marah. It says here that they murmured against Moses, saying, 'What shall we drink?' (15:24). Moses cried to the Lord, and the Lord showed him a tree. When he cast it into the waters, the waters were made sweet. Then it says, 'There He made for them a statute and an ordinance for them, and there He tested them and said, "If you diligently heed the voice of the Lord your God and do what is right in His sight, give ear to His commandments, and keep all His statutes, I will put none of the diseases on you which I have brought on the Egyptians. For I am the Lord who heals you"' (vv. 15–26)."

Looking up from her copy of Scripture, Karla asked, "Is this what they were telling you about?"

"That's it," Liz replied. "So do you think it means what they say it did?"

"Well, first of all, I certainly don't want to put your sister or her husband down—or their church. I have a number of friends who view this passage, and others, the way they do. But I'm really convinced, Liz—and I've talked at length with our pastor about this as well—that we can't always equate cancer or some serious disease with God's judgment for a specific sin. Nor can we say it's always God's will to heal us if we just have enough faith. Part of the reason for that is in this very passage. Part of it comes from some verses in the New Testament. But do you feel up to this discussion right now?"

> *Sickness, decay, and death are a*
> *direct consequence of the rebellion of*
> *our first parents against God.*

"Sure," Liz smiled. "Besides if I get this resolved in my mind, it will probably help me rest easier—and maybe even cope with having cancer better. I still feel overwhelmed a lot of the time, even hopeless. Bill's been a tower of strength, but I sense he's pretty frightened about all this too."

Sin and Sickness

The viewpoint Liz picked up from her sister and brother-in-law is an extremely common way of understanding the connection between sickness and sin. As we noted in an earlier chapter, questions about sickness and sin, and about sickness and faith, have been around ever since Job's friends encouraged him to confess the evil they were convinced was lurking in his heart, ever since the disciples voiced the question to Jesus about whose sin caused the disability of the man who was born blind (Job 4:7; John 9:2–3).

Frequently sin and sickness are directly linked. One example is Jesus' healing of the paralytic (Mark 2:3–12); another is Paul's discussion about physical illness resulting from mishandling the Lord's Supper in Corinth (1 Corinthians 11:29–30). Yet there are two important truths we must hold in balance. One is the connection between all physical and emotional illness and the Fall. A careful examination of Genesis 1–3 reveals that sickness, decay, and death are a direct consequence of the rebellion of our first parents against God. In that sense, every instance of illness, every cancer, every heart attack, is linked to sin.

However, the balancing truth on the other side of the equation is that not every instance of physical illness is connected with some specific personal sin—or even a deficiency in personal faith. The apostle Paul, a gifted healer of others (Acts 28:8–9), unsuccessfully sought God's healing on at least three occasions (see chapter 3). And Jesus made clear that no specific sin of the man born blind (that would have been ludicrous, since his condition existed from birth), or of his parents, caused his blindness. Rather, his inability to see was designed to glorify Jesus as the Light of the World, the one who provides true sight.

WHAT ABOUT JEHOVAH RAPHA?

But what about passages such as the one from which Liz raised the question concerning Jehovah Rapha? Throughout the Old Testament, various names for God were given to focus our attention on His person and help us understand some facet of His character. An examination of these passages in context can help us understand what the authors of Scripture were seeking to convey about God's character, provide encouragement for us when we face difficulty, disease, or even the consequences of disobedience, and help us guard against the danger of misunderstanding or misapplying Scripture.

The first of these titles, Jehovah Jireh, is found in Genesis 22:14, where Abraham is offering his son Isaac as an act of obedience and dedication to God. In response to a question from his vigorous, strapping young son, Abraham voiced confident faith in the Lord's ability to provide a substitute sacrifice. Understanding and accepting his father's faith, Isaac freely submitted to him. The ultimate confidence in God expressed by both was rewarded when, as Abraham was in the very act of lifting the knife to take his son's life, God interrupted to call the patriarch's attention to a substitute ram caught in a nearby thicket.

The second of these titles, Jehovah Rapha, appears in Exodus 15:26, the passage under discussion by Liz and Karla. It and the next title—Jehovah Nissi, the Lord our banner (Exodus

17:15)—both appear in the narrative description of Israel's deliverance from Egypt and the journey toward the promised land.

In the first incident, God provides healthy drinking water when only polluted water was present, preventing the kind of serious illnesses the Israelites had seen the Egyptians experience as a result of the ten plagues. In the second incident, the people of Israel were under attack by the Amalekites. Though God supernaturally provided victory through the upraised rod in the hand of Moses, it was still necessary for the Israelite soldiers to fight against the Amalekites under the direction of Joshua.

It isn't enough simply to claim God's healing, rebuke Satan the enemy, or sit back hoping for an instant miracle.

These two incidents, found in close proximity in the Old Testament, teach a common important lesson—the balance between dependence on God and human initiative. Whereas Jehovah Rapha provided clean, pure water, Moses had to cut down a tree at God's direction, then cast it into the waters of this wilderness oasis. Whereas Jehovah Nissi provided the banner of victory for the Israelites, the leadership skills of Joshua and the individual efforts of each Israelite soldier played an essential part of the divine plan for victory.

These two incidents hold great practical significance for Christians who face cancer and other dreaded diseases today. It isn't enough simply to claim God's healing, rebuke Satan the enemy, or sit back hoping for an instant miracle. Time after time, throughout Scripture and in our modern era as well, God has utilized a combination we have chosen to label "active waiting" on the Lord. Active waiting includes the three components we identified in chapter 3. The first is an absolute confidence in God's ability to heal, expressed in believing prayer. The second is a willingness to vigorously pursue the best available medical care, plus personal efforts to strengthen and care for our physical bodies. The third is a total trust both in God's goodness and in His sovereignty, no matter what happens.

Throughout Scripture the concept of waiting is both encouraged and exemplified. The lips of the patriarch Jacob confess, "I have waited for your salvation, O Lord" (Genesis 49:18); the apostle Paul writes to urge believers to wait for His son from heaven (1 Thessalonians 1:10). This concept is often extolled as an ideal Christian virtue. However, it is also important to recognize that Jacob wrestled with the Angel of the Lord (Genesis 32:24), whereas the apostle Paul pointed out to New Testament Christians that those who engaged in waiting without involvement in personal responsibility were not to be allowed to eat (2 Thessalonians 3:10–11).

OTHER NAMES FOR GOD

In other portions of the Old Testament, the authors of Scripture used additional titles for God—titles that have come to signify some valuable aspect of His character and attitude toward us. Psalm 23, perhaps the most familiar and best-loved passage in the Old Testament, begins with the title Jehovah Roeh, the Lord my shepherd. Anyone who understands the culture of David's day and the total, compassionate care a shepherd gave each of his sheep can grasp what this title communicated to the Israelites about their personal God and His care for them.

Another title, Jehovah Shalom—the Lord our peace—appears against the backdrop of the darkest, most conflict-filled days in Israel—the time of the judges. The nation had disobeyed God, and He permitted the people to suffer the consequences of oppression at the hand of a hostile tribe called the Midianites. During these bleak days the Angel of the Lord appeared to Gideon, whose question about his people's troubles provides a remarkable parallel to the questions voiced by Liz and others with cancer: "If the Lord is with us, why then has all this happened to us? And where are all His miracles which our fathers told us about. . . . But now the Lord has forsaken us and delivered us into the hands of the Midianites" (Judges 6:13).

At this point the preincarnate Christ—the Angel of the Lord—looked at Gideon and said, "Go in this might of yours and you shall save Israel from the hand of the Midianites. Have I not sent you?" (v. 14). In response to Gideon's protest of weakness, the Lord promises to be with him, accepts his offered sacrifice, then miraculously consumes the sacrifice as a sign to Gideon.

When Gideon realizes that he is actually face to face with the Angel of the Lord, he reacts with fear, since he recognizes that to look on the face of God could bring death. Immediately the Lord reassures him: "Peace be with you; do not fear, you shall not die" (v. 23). In response, Gideon builds an altar, naming it for the God of peace, Jehovah Shalom. For us today the peace provided through Christ makes possible a right relationship with God through forgiveness of sins (Ephesians 2:14–15). It is His peace that sustains us in times of great trouble and seasons of inner anxiety (Philippians 4:6–7).

The final title is found in the very last verse of Ezekiel. Looking ahead to the millennial reign of the Messiah in the gloriously rebuilt city of David, the prophet refers to the city as Jehovah Shammah—the Lord is there. Against a panorama of sin, failure, and abandonment by God, Ezekiel directs his Israelite contemporaries' attention ahead in glorious hope to a magnificent city—but, more important, a city characterized by the presence of God.

For Liz and others facing the perplexing questions—the whys, the wherefores, "Why me?" "Why now?" "What's going on?" and "Where is God?"—that seem to descend like a swarm of bees to sting the minds of those with cancer, the very first place to focus is on the person of God. Not on circumstances, not even on the issue of a cure—the place to begin to deal with the *spiritual* component of such a debilitating illness is with the goodness and power of God. That's precisely where Karla sought to focus Liz's attention when her friend voiced concerns about what she had heard from her sister and brother-in-law.

Back to Liz and Karla

"Let's take a look at who's doing the talking in Exodus 15 and who He's talking to," Karla suggested. "Verses 22–25 describe what happen. Then, beginning in verse 26, we have God's instruction to Moses. You know, I'm pretty sure your sister and brother-in-law are not right in applying this to you. To be honest, based on what we've learned in our Bible study, it seems pretty straightforward to interpret this as a promise God made to Israel in the context of His setting them free from Egypt. Take a look at this."

Rising from her seat, Karla placed her copy of Scripture where Liz could see it. "See what it says? 'There He made a statute and an ordinance for them. And there He tested them'— right there in verse 25, just before He calls Himself the Lord who heals you." Taking a ballpoint pen from her purse, Karla underscored both uses of the word "them."

Nodding, Liz looked up from the page of the Bible in front of her. "What you say sure seems consistent with the way we were taught to interpret Scripture in our Bible study. Always look at who's talking and to whom. In fact, look here. Verse 26 is specifically addressed to Israel. '[If *you* obey,] I will put none of the diseases on you which I have brought on the Egyptians.'"

As Karla nodded her head, Liz sighed deeply. "Well, it sure would be nice to be able to say we know that God's will is always to heal us. My sister seemed so certain about that. She kept talking about all the people Jesus healed in the New Testament and about the verse in Isaiah 53. You know, 'By His stripes we are healed.'"

Both good and bad things happen to both good and bad people.

Karla looked at her friend without saying anything for a moment. "I've wondered about that verse too. So I asked our pastor about it one day. He explained that the context of Isaiah 53 is a discussion about transgressions and iniquities—about *spiritual* sickness—sickness of the soul, he called it. He told me that, even though Jesus healed a lot of people during His ministry, there were far more He did *not* heal. Those He did heal were for a purpose, to show who He was—Messiah and God. He also said that His healing of physical diseases sort of anticipated His healing the bigger problem of sin through His death on the cross, and that's what Isaiah had in mind."

Karla paused, noticing that her friend was nodding off. "Tell you what, Liz. I know this is a pretty tiring discussion. Suppose we continue it another time."

"Can you come back tomorrow?" Liz asked. "I'm sure that tomorrow morning I'll feel a lot more rested. Maybe I won't have taken this pain medication. It just makes me get sleepy all of a sudden sometimes."

"Tell you what I'll do," Karla suggested. "Let me take a look at some things tonight. There's something in the back of my mind about Job and about Paul that may shed some light on what we're talking about. But before I go, why don't we pray together?"

Understanding Sickness

The conversation between Liz and her friend Karla is not unusual. Perhaps it would be helpful to summarize several observations regarding illnesses such as cancer before we rejoin Karla for another visit with Liz.

1 *Whereas sickness is a consequence of the Fall, sickness does not always correspond with unrighteousness or a specific sin*. Jesus articulated a general principle during the Sermon on the Mount whereby He urged His listeners to love their enemies (Matthew 5:44). The principle is simple: The Father "makes His sun rise on the evil and on the good, and sends rain on the just and on the unjust" (v. 45). Jesus' point is that both good and bad things happen to both good and bad people. Human experience has shown time and again that disasters don't always happen to those who, in our judgment, richly deserve them. Nor do those who live just lives always escape the consequences, physical and otherwise, of living in a fallen environment.

One classic example of this principle is Job. Described in Scripture as an upright man who feared God and shunned evil, this patriarch was severely tested by a series of personal crises that included the loss of his children and his vast financial holdings (see chapter 3). What a simple yet profound lesson for us! Sickness will come. Adversity will happen. There will be sunny days and stormy times. And though it is important for us to examine our hearts whenever sickness occurs to be sure that there is not some unresolved issue of hidden sin (1 Corinthians 11:31), it is equally important not to jump to the conclusion that either our sickness or that of someone else has been caused directly by sin or a lack of faith.

2 *It is important to view physical health as a "good gift from God."* The apostle James reminds us that "every good gift and every perfect gift is from above, and comes down from the Father of lights, with whom there is no variation or shadow of turning" (James 1:17). Two implications are clear from this principle. First, I am to live a life of thankfulness for whatever health and strength I have. Frequently, as we saw in the responses of the families of some who were hospitalized, along with Jessica Eggert (chapter 3), some loudly lament their circumstances without recognizing that others may be far worse off than they. Well spoken is the old proverb about the man who complained because he had no shoes until he met another man who had no feet.

There is a second implication of this principle: Not only am I to thank God for my health, I am to treasure that health by taking care of myself. A later chapter will have more to say about preventing cancer—avoiding carcinogens, eating appropriately, exercising consistently, and other steps we can take to maintain our health. Yet the principle is clear. Guarding what we have and taking care of what we have been given are both important and appropriate responses to the God who graciously gives.

3 *Although sickness was not part of God's original plan, He can and will use sickness just as He uses other circumstances in our lives.* Two classic examples stand out in Scripture—Job in the Old Testament, Paul in the New. There is no question that Job's series of disasters tested him to the extreme. Even James reminded his readers, "You have heard of the perseverance of Job" (James 5:11).

Ironically, although Job was acknowledged as a man of incredible spiritual stature, there was within the inner recesses of his being a weakness, a fear. It was only after his final disaster occurred that Job acknowledged that what he had feared most had come to pass (Job 3:25). Recognizing his own inability to see God through the fog of his circumstances, he acknowledged, "But He knows the way that I take. When He has tested me, I shall come forth as gold" (Job 23:10).

Through the pain of his illness and his multiple adversities, Job had become convinced that God had His eye upon him every step of the way—much as David confessed in Psalm

32:8. Furthermore, God had allowed these circumstances—including the illness and its consequences—as a part of a test, a test with a gracious and positive purpose.

Job further acknowledged three important principles that allowed God's purpose to be fulfilled through the patriarch's adversity. First, he was committed to obeying God, to walking in close fellowship with Him: "My foot has held fast to His steps; I have kept His way and not turned aside" (Job 23:11). During times of illness and despair we may often be tempted to turn away from God in bitter rebellion. As one man once put it, "If God can't treat me any better than this—if He's going to make my life miserable—I'll just go out and enjoy life as much as I can." Such an attitude was far from the mind of Job.

Second, the patriarch kept his thinking straight by making God's word a priority during his adversity. "I have not departed from the commandment of His lips; I have treasured the words of His mouth more than my necessary food" (Job 23:12). For Job, the key to spiritual strength during his time of great physical adversity was to continue meditating (mentally feasting) on the word of God. During a period of national disaster, the prophet Jeremiah had much the same experience: "Your words were found, and I ate them, and Your word was to me the joy and rejoicing of my heart; for I am called by Your name, O Lord God of Hosts" (Jeremiah 15:16).

A third principle God taught Job during this time of testing was the importance of recognizing and resting in the unparalleled sovereignty of God: "But He is unique, and who can make Him change? And whatever His soul desires, that He does" (Job 23:13). Recognizing that God is both absolutely sovereign and intrinsically good, Job responds in awe with what other biblical writers refer to as "the fear of the Lord"—a submissive, reverential trust.

For Paul, as for Job, sickness was not a direct consequence of some specific sin (see chapter 3). Often, sickness *is* the result of sinful behavior, but in such cases the sin is usually obvious. For example, the risk of cancer of the cervix has been shown by research to have a direct correlation to the number of sexual partners a person has had. Many studies have proven lung cancer to be a common consequence of abusing the body by smoking. And research on AIDS has documented the connection, in many cases, between immoral sexual practices or forms of drug abuse and contracting the illness. Yet it is important not to make generalizations in other cases, as Liz's sister and brother-in-law tended to do or as Job's friends did.

In Paul's case, God allowed some physical adversity, described by the apostle as "a thorn in the flesh," to come into his life. We are not suggesting that Paul suffered from some form of cancer, although that seems within the realm of possibility. He could have experienced some chronic malady such as ophthalmia, malaria, migraine headaches, or even epilepsy.[1] But Paul wasn't hung up over the details of his physical diagnosis. He looked beyond that to see what spiritual point this thorn carried. Ironically, in Paul's case, it seems that there were two totally opposite purposes, being sought by God and Satan respectively, through the same set of adverse circumstances.

> *Whereas some things are not good in and of themselves, good can be gained from every situation—even physical illness, financial disaster, or the tragedy of abuse.*

Paul first acknowledges that God had a purpose, a good and positive design, in his adversity. This purpose was preventive in nature: "lest I should be exalted above measure by the abundance of the revelations" (2 Corinthians 12:7). A loving God sensed a possibly dangerous weakness in the life of His choice servant and allowed the experience of adversity to meet that need.

In the case of Job, the weakness seemed to be fear—an inability to trust God. In Paul's case, the weakness was a tendency toward pride—toward self-reliance rather than utter dependence upon God. After all, the apostle had identified himself to the Philippians as a Pharisee of the Pharisees. Pharisees were religiously the most self-reliant people of that day. Yet Paul had renounced his pharisaic heritage, choosing to trust Christ and humbly walk with Him. In 2 Corinthians 10:1, he underscores his own gentleness and humility: "Now I, Paul, myself, am pleading with you by the meekness and gentleness of Christ—who in presence am lowly among you, but being absent am bold toward you."

And as every individual who has strapped on football gear or every person who has laced up basketball sneakers for serious competition or every person who has ever run a mile or utilized a StairMaster® or a NordicTrack® has learned, there is truly no gain without pain. The goal for the Christian is to determine precisely the direction and nature of God's intended gain, then joyfully endure the pain. Gary Smalley refers to this as *treasure hunting.*

Treasure Hunting

During his frequent appearances with his colleague John Trent on our radio talk show "Life Perspectives," Gary often encourages those who are experiencing physical or emotional adversity to engage in treasure hunting. Gary is convinced of the promise of Romans 8:28 that, whereas some things are not good in and of themselves, good can be gained from every situation—even physical illness, financial disaster, or the tragedy of abuse. Gary has penned memorable words to explain how this treasure-hunting principle works: "Every problem—great or small—has in it a treasure waiting to be discovered. The secret to successful treasure hunting is understanding two life-changing words: faith and love."[2]

Developing an absolute trust in God and a genuine compassion toward people, these are among the positive results of "treasure hunting." On a number of these radio programs, Gary has candidly discussed a situation about which he writes in *Joy That Lasts.* The occasion involves an extended conflict with a colleague. It was a trying time for Gary, one that seemed to produce only negative emotions and circumstances. Yet ultimately, through this conflict and its resolution, Gary came to a stronger love and appreciation for his wife and family, an extended ministry opportunity involving a nationwide seminar ministry, the writing of best-selling books on marriage and parenting, and numerous opportunities to counsel and encourage through personal contact and radio ministries.

Seated in a coffee shop in suburban Dallas late one evening at the close of a hectic day, eating pancakes with colleague John Trent and a ministry friend, Gary's eyes lit up when the subject of treasure hunting was brought up.

"I didn't like the idea, to be frank about it. It grew out of one of the worst experiences of my life. But God had to teach me that the world's viewpoint—that suffering is bad and must be avoided whenever possible—is wrong, wrong, wrong! A good example of this is my friend Monte Johnson. Monte was an all-pro linebacker for the Raiders. But when he tore up the cartilage in his knee, things looked hopeless for his football career. So he and I sat down together to talk about how the knee injury and the prospect of his release from the Raiders might become a benefit. Monte came up with a number of benefits that would come his way. If he were cut by the Raiders, he would have more time with his family. He might even have an opportunity to go into a ministry.

"That's exactly what happened. In fact, Monte really shocked the coach who told him he had been cut because his knee was no longer strong enough to support a career in pro football when he said, 'I thank God for using you to help me discover what God wants me to do with the rest of my life.'

"So Monte became involved with a respected Christian financial counseling and management program designed to help athletes and other professionals plan for the future. And he was able to find even more time to spend with his family than he did during his career in professional sports."

This experience of Monte Johnson, described by Gary Smalley, is a classic example of how God can utilize physical weakness and pain to produce spiritual benefit. For Monte it was a physical injury, for Gary a personal conflict, for Paul a "thorn in the flesh," for Job a series of disasters, and for Liz lung cancer. Yet in each situation, God was at work to produce something good, positive, and spiritually beneficial.

Liz Understands

Karla was bubbling with excitement as she entered Liz's room the next morning; she spoke pleasantly to the nurse who was just leaving, then greeted her friend warmly with a hug. She noted with a smile the open window, the curtains pulled back, and the summer sunshine that seemed to flood the room.

"You seem to feel better today—did you rest well last night?"

"Sure did," Liz replied. "And I've really been looking forward to hearing what you have to share with me today."

Removing the maroon Bible from her handbag, Karla snapped it open and flipped to the place she had already marked. "Second Corinthians 12," she announced—"Paul's thorn in the flesh."

Karla shared with Liz the truths already discussed in this chapter. Then she said, "I think Satan wanted Paul to suffer—to the point even of giving up. I went back and read 2 Corinthians all the way through last night. Twice I noticed that Paul said, 'We do not lose heart.' He was hard-pressed on every side, but not crushed. Perplexed, but not despairing. Persecuted, but not forsaken. Struck down, but not destroyed. Liz, I bet Satan wanted Paul to give up—or at least, to be shaken. But God wanted to strengthen him, to strengthen the hidden flaw of pride in his life."

Karla paused for a moment to pull her chair closer to the bed. "Do you remember that disaster back in the early eighties in Kansas City, at the Hyatt Regency Hotel?"

"You mean those sky bridges that collapsed?"

"Right. Over one hundred people died—and that building was practically new! But they found out later that there were hidden flaws in the design and manufacture of the steel bolts that held those sky bridges in place. Liz, I lost some close friends there—they died when those skywalks collapsed. If someone had found the hidden flaws, it might not have happened."

"So you're saying that God may allow things like sickness and pain—even cancer—to help strengthen hidden flaws in our lives?"

"I think that's what happened to Paul, and even to Job in the Old Testament. Remember, he admitted after all those terrible things happened that he had struggled with fear all along."

"So Job had a hidden weakness—fear. Paul had a weakness too—a tendency toward pride."

"Exactly. God graciously allowed their suffering as a means of strengthening them against spiritual disaster." Karla noticed a puzzled expression on the face of her friend.

"But does that mean we shouldn't pray to get well?"

"Absolutely not," Karla countered. "Paul said he pleaded with the Lord three times for relief. But God told him, 'My grace is sufficient for you, for My strength is made perfect in weakness.'"

"So let me see if I can put this all together—what we talked about yesterday and today. Cancer and other kinds of sickness are a result of the Fall."

"Right. Just like cancer cells infect a person's body, sin has infected the human race. Cancer and other forms of sickness are just one of the results."

"But not every sickness is a consequence of a specific sin?"

"Right again. Some are, like the Corinthians who abused their communion love feast. But some, like the man Jesus healed who had been born blind, clearly aren't."

The option to relieve or not to relieve suffering or sickness rests completely with the God who is too good to do us wrong and too powerful not to be in control.

"So I need to examine my heart for unconfessed sin but not worry that some sin I don't know about has caused my sickness."

"Exactly," Karla responded. "I think if we walk in obedience to God's word and feed ourselves regularly on Scripture, God will make us aware of hidden sin in our lives."

"But we *should* look for whatever good purpose God may be trying to accomplish—or weakness He may be using the sickness to strengthen."

"Precisely. And I think it's appropriate to pray for relief from pain—and even from the sickness. At times God *does* answer that prayer affirmatively. He has healed many people, even from cancer—the doctors call it spontaneous remission. But more commonly, I believe God chooses to work through a combination of trust in the sovereignty of God and a sort of active waiting on the Lord. The kind of waiting that prays for relief but can also recognize that, as Paul put it, 'When I am weak, then I am strong'" (2 Corinthians 12:10).

Practical Perspectives

As creatures who are susceptible to extremes, cancer patients frequently take one of a number of unbalanced approaches. Some insist on a miracle, an immediate cure. We agree that it is appropriate to pray like the apostle Paul did, to ask God for relief. But we also urge recognition that the option to relieve or not to relieve suffering or sickness rests completely with the God who is too good to do us wrong and too powerful not to be in control.

Another unbalanced approach is to fatalistically give up. Those who do this often view cancer as a curse, a judgment from God, even a death sentence. Such an approach is both unbiblical and unrealistic.

Finally, some individuals—even Christians—take a rationalistic, humanistic approach. They seek the best medical care but without prayer—they ignore the dimension of trusting God.

James strongly urged a balanced approach, one that included both the spiritual resource of prayer and human encouragement and support. Those who were suffering were to pray (James 5:13). Those who were ill—the term James uses means to be weak or weary and can indicate physical, emotional, or even spiritual weaknesses—were to call for the elders of the church. They were to initiate two activities: praying over the ill person and anointing him or her with oil.

Whereas there are those who practice and encourage a ceremony of anointing sick people with oil (and we have seen encouragement and benefit from this), the term James uses for *anoint* is not the common New Testament word for ceremonial anointing. Instead, the apostle employs another word, which means "to rub or pour" with oil—as a host would do in welcoming an honored guest in the culture of that day (Luke 7:46) or as a person would do, along with washing the face, to avoid giving a sad appearance as part of the grooming process (Matthew 6:17). Other commentators have interpreted the use of oil in James as descriptive of seeking good medical care, recognizing the "well-documented fact that oil was one of the most common medicines of biblical times."[3]

In summary, it seems that this passage does not rule out a ceremony of anointing with oil. However, its primary point is to urge Christians to take action to encourage the weak and discouraged by providing a physical and a spiritual uplift, which can lead to spiritual and emotional restoration.

But is James's promised restoration physical or spiritual? As one commentator notes, "Many physically ill Christians have called on elders to pray for them and to anoint them with oil. But a sizable percentage of them have remained sick. This fact suggests that the passage may have been mistakenly understood as physical restoration, rather than spiritual restoration."[4]

Whereas it is clear that it is not always God's will to heal an illness, it is always His purpose to use godly individuals to provide spiritual encouragement and help restore uplifting hope to those who are weak and in despair. After all, since Christians are the only individuals promised hope beyond this life (1 Corinthians 15:19–22), God wants us to be walking in hope no matter how grim our physical circumstances. On a practical level what should our approach be?

First, face the future with absolute trust in God. Even though Satan, disease, and death are among our enemies, God is for us—so who can stand against us (Romans 8:31)?

Second, reach out to God in prayer. The emphasis of James's exhortation to those who were weak was toward prayer. The elders were to pray (James 5:14), the individual was to pray (v. 15), and the church as a whole was to pray (v. 16). James concludes his remarks with a reminder that "the effective, fervent prayer of a righteous man avails much" (v. 16).

Third, reach out for support. James encourages the individual weakened by sickness to call for the elders, then urges the entire church to "confess your trespasses to one another, and pray for one another, that you may be healed" (v. 16). All too often Christians adopt what we earlier referred to as the "lone ranger" mentality. There are far too many "one anothers" in Scripture to allow for such an approach.

Fourth, avoid the extremes. Don't fall into the trap of insisting that God perform a miracle for you right now. The Bible is not the Arabian Nights, and God is not Aladdin's genie, popping out of a lamp to grant three wishes as part of a Disney production. Nor is He an uncaring, uninvolved sovereign. So neither should we simply give up or even pursue medical care apart from the spiritual resources of prayer or God's word.

We strongly urge the combination we have labeled "active waiting"—doing everything that is our responsibility to do —from seeking good medical treatment to taking care of our bodies—while leaving everything outside our control to God and those, such as medical professionals, who are trained and equipped to deal with those things.

Fifth, learn to live one day at a time. That was the approach Paul took in 2 Corinthians 4:16–17. Even in the process of anticipating ultimate physical death, he recognized the importance of living life one day at a time.

Finally, look for the treasure. Seek to determine—through prayer, time in the Word, and the counsel of other individuals —just what God is seeking to teach you, what He wants to strengthen regarding your walk with Him. Perhaps, as in the case of Job, He is seeking to uproot hidden fear. Or, like Paul, you may need an extra dose of humility.

Whatever the case, recognize that He has a gracious and good purpose, one consistent with the hope to which He has called you. As Paul reminds us, we can rejoice in tribulations, knowing they produce perseverance, lead to approved character, and ultimately result in a hope that does not disappoint (Romans 5:3–5). We can rest with confidence in the reminder of the prophet Jeremiah, written during days of captivity, adversity, sickness, and death:

> For I know the thoughts that I think toward you, says the Lord, thoughts of peace and not of evil, to give you a future and a hope. Then you will call upon Me and go and pray to Me, and I will listen to you. And you will seek Me and find Me when you search for Me with all your heart." (Jeremiah 29:11–13)

8

TREATING CANCER

For Tom (see chapter 1), the best option for dealing with his prostate cancer proved to be right across town—M.D. Anderson Hospital in Houston. For Candy (see chapter 6), another internationally respected facility—the Mayo Clinic—provided resources for treating the cancer that invaded her head. These facilities, plus Memorial Sloan-Kettering Cancer Center in New York, Oschner's in New Orleans, and a few others are ranked among the most respected cancer research and treatment centers in the world.

But like thousands of others who have been diagnosed with cancer, Cliff (see chapter 3) simply chose to have his treatment take place in the best available facility where he lived. Tall in stature and of athletic build, Cliff had lost significant weight because of the tumor in his colon. Now he and his wife sat in the office of his oncologist, Dr. Horace Short, who had been recommended by the kindly, silver-haired Dr. Paul Handley who had treated Cliff's father before him. Cliff thought, *I've certainly received a lot of advice from friends and relatives. But these are the two men I plan to trust with my treatment.*

Reaching over to squeeze Gloria's hand, Cliff smiled at his wife, then turned his attention to the two physicians sitting across the room from them. "You guys are my main men. My go-to guys," Cliff said, alluding to basketball, a sport he had played regularly ever since his own days in junior high school. "Horace, as I see it you're my point guard—the guy who'll call the plays on the court, then make sure they're executed proper-ly. And you, Dr. Handley—well, you're the dean of coaches. You've been the medical coach for our family for three genera-tions now. Since I'm the middle generation, I'm putting my life in your hands—at least humanly speaking.

"However, before you guys tell me what's ahead for me regarding treatment, I want you to know that my ultimate confi-dence is in the Great Physician. Gloria and I are more strongly committed to our faith in Christ than ever before. I know God has some good purpose for me in this cancer, as well as some tough lessons. Like you told me the other day, Dr. Handley, it could get me—statistically, the odds are it will.

"But I teach history to college students. Over the years I've seen that history sometimes takes an unexpected turn. Mir-acles do happen. They're often the result of prayer, dedication, and hard work. Gloria and I have asked a network of our family and closest friends to pray for us every day—and to pray for you men and the rest of the treatment team."

Pausing, Cliff noticed a smile on the face of Dr. Handley. Dr. Short, on the other hand, was frowning. His voice carried a note of irritation. "Frankly, Cliff, I'm not real big on religion. I've had some patients who seemed to use it as a cop-out—didn't really follow through on their treatment—just sort of left every-thing in the hands of God. I believe God helps those who help themselves. That's what good cancer care is all about. Helping yourself with the best available treatment, then developing a positive attitude.

"Now don't get me wrong. I'm not saying that religion it-self will hurt a person. Only when they allow it to get in the way of good medical care. The same thing with overdoing this posi-tive thinking business—you know, guided imagery and all that New Age stuff. I met a patient here recently who dropped out right in the middle of radiotherapy. Told me he picked up a book that told him all he had to do was think positive and he'd be able to lick his cancer. Something about just visualizing all his white blood cells surrounding all the cancer cells—sort of a Star Wars of the bloodstream." Dr. Short paused and self-con-sciously rubbed his balding head. "To be honest, I think a positive attitude helps, but there are a lot of things in the body that you just can't control with positive thinking."

With a quick sidewise glance at his wife, Cliff replied, "I think I hear where you're coming from, Dr. Short. Thanks for your candor. To be honest with you, I couldn't agree more about the positive thinking or New Age approach. A few years ago I broke my leg in a pickup basketball game—had to use crutches for almost a year. Now, I'm as positive a thinker as they come—my wife will attest to that. But no amount of positive thinking could cause that bone in my leg to heal any quicker or better, or put me back on the court before the break had time to heal."

Dr. Short's frown had been replaced by a smile. As he nodded vigorously, Cliff continued. "Now, about this matter of religion. I guess you could say I see that the same way too. I don't put a lot of stock in religion. I see trying to be religious to please God as kinda like a man with cancer trying to treat himself. I suspect, Dr. Short, that if you were diagnosed with cancer, you probably wouldn't treat yourself—even though you're a cancer specialist." Both physicians nodded.

"You'd want to get someone who was skilled, but who could be objective in designing a treatment plan for you that would work. That's how I view the matter of faith. Instead of trying to be religious and earn God's favor myself, I realize that I was infected with a sort of spiritual cancer, with no ability to cure myself. That's why I placed my trust in Jesus Christ. He actually took care of the root of my problem Himself by dying in my place. So now I trust Him for everything—including what I'm facing because I have cancer." The frown had returned to Dr. Short's face.

"That doesn't mean that I exercise blind faith without good medical care. It's like the day my son Roger and I went fishing. Last summer we were out on a little lake in a rowboat and a storm blew up. So we did two things: We prayed hard to God for safety—and we rowed hard to shore to find shelter. Guess you could say that's my motto, Doc. Pray hard and row to shore."

Dr. Short replied reluctantly, "OK, Cliff. I think I understand where you're coming from. So let's get down to your specific treatment program."

I suspect Dr. Short and I may clash over the course of this treatment at some point, Cliff thought. *I want to do everything I can to avoid that—but I'm sure not going to compromise my faith in the process.*

Getting the News

Cliff thought back over the traumatic events of recent days. Nearing fifty, he had been in the blush of health for many years, with the exception of a few colds, occasional allergy problems, and the broken leg he had mentioned to Dr. Short. During his forties, he had struggled with a tendency to put on weight—a struggle compounded by his fondness for rare steaks and chocolates. "I've been diagnosed as a chocaholic," he used to tell his friends. "After all, I consider chocolate one of the four basic food groups—and even occasionally lie awake at night worrying about a world chocolate shortage. So I must be addicted."

However, over the previous six months, Cliff had begun losing weight without even trying. Concerned, Gloria had urged him to get a checkup. Dr. Handley, who had done the initial checkup, suggested X rays of the gastrointestinal tract—"a lower GI" he had called it. Cliff remembered joking with Dr. Handley. "I can't have one of those. I was in the navy. I never was a GI!"

"So what's the treatment, Doc— and what's my prognosis? Can we lick this thing, or is it likely to kill me?"

Cliff remembered the laxatives and enemas, the horrible taste of the barium—that was for the "upper GI"—then the barium enema, administered under the supervision of a radiologist—a tight-lipped man who had refused to give Cliff even a clue about what he had seen.

Cliff's thoughts flashed back to the day following the tests, when he had sat in one of the uncomfortable chairs in Dr. Handley's office and learned about the golfball-sized tumor located about fifteen inches up from the bottom of his colon.

"There it is," Dr. Handley had said, pointing to the X ray in his hand. "There's the reason for your weight loss, Cliff. It's the second most common cancer in the United States—but nobody likes to talk about it very much. It actually was ranked first before lung cancer became so common. Yours is located in what we call the sigmoid colon—sigmoid means curved—just below the descending colon. You may not have known this, Cliff, but you actually have an ascending, a transverse, and a descending colon, in addition to your sigmoid colon."

"Maybe if I taught English instead of history I'd see a little more humor in my situation," Cliff responded, trying to break through the shock of the news he had just received. "So what's the treatment, Doc—and what's my prognosis? Can we lick this thing, or is it likely to kill me?"

"It all depends, Cliff. The overall average prognosis for colon cancer is approximately 50 percent—much higher than that if it is a localized Stage One cancer, but less than 10 percent for cancers that have spread."

Choosing Your Treatment Team

Cliff remembered Dr. Handley's pointed instruction: "The first thing you need to do is pick the doctor and the place for your treatment. The oncologist—the cancer specialist—comes first. Choosing your primary care doctor is actually more crucial than picking a specific hospital. At least that's the way I view things."

Cliff recalled raising the issue of being treated at one of the nationally known cancer locations. "Sure that's an option," Dr. Handley had replied. "But the National Cancer Institute has an information service that gives doctors all over the country a computerized report on the latest treatment protocol for any patient's specific kind and stage of cancer. You can even call one of the experts and talk to them yourself if you'd like to do so."

Cliff and Dr. Handley had talked at length before the two of them agreed on the choice of Dr. Short as oncologist. In most typical situations, a cancer patient will have a primary care physician—often the family practice doctor who is already your personal physician, who knows you and may have even served your family. However, our highly mobile society has left many families and individuals with no relationship to a family practice doctor. Many people bypass regular checkups and only go to hospital emergency rooms or suburban emergency care clinics when treatment is needed. Though such facilities meet a growing need in our society, we still encourage healthy people to cultivate a relationship with a family doctor or personal physician.

The primary care physician will work closely with the other leading member of the treatment team—the oncologist, who is a physician trained in the causes and treatments of various forms of cancer. The primary care physician and the oncologist are usually not proficient at surgical procedures, so often a surgeon is called in to perform necessary operations. Radiologists are involved both in the diagnosis of cancer—utilizing magnetic resonance imaging (MRI), CAT scan (computerized axial tomography), ultrasound, and X rays to show in vivid detail precisely what is taking place with the tumor—and in radiotherapy.

Cliff recalled being given a local anesthetic, then having an eight-inch needle inserted into a spot marked carefully at a precise location on his abdomen. Cells taken from the spot were delivered to a pathologist, who placed them on a glass slide, then carefully examined the individual cells under a strong microscope. His diagnosis: a malignant neoplasm of the sigmoid colon—the most common kind and location of colon cancer.

The colon cancer diagnosed today typically is found in polyps that have taken perhaps ten or twenty years, even more, to develop. President Ronald Reagan was diagnosed with a fairly large (5 cm) malignant polyp, which was successfully removed in 1985 following a diagnostic sigmoidoscopy, an examination of the colon through a tube inserted in the rectum. Cliff's physician had considered a sigmoidoscopy, but instead had opted for the more extensive upper and lower GI series of tests.

The Physician-Patient Relationship

Our experience has taught us that an effective working relationship—in effect, a partnership—is essential for successfully treating any form of cancer. Thus the choice of a physician for cancer care becomes crucial.

In our judgment, there are three essentials: the doctor must have appropriate skills and knowledge, a genuine care for patients, and a willingness to communicate. We have seen many instances where excellent medical skills were rendered less than effective by an uncaring attitude or an unwillingness to communicate.

It is important to remember that, no matter how competent the physician you choose, you are ultimately your own patient advocate.

One way to evaluate a prospective doctor is to talk both with former patients and with medical colleagues if at all possible. Sometimes information can be secured from a local medical society. Even the local library can provide a list of specialists. Board certification is another way to determine the expertise of a physician. When a doctor has become board certified, he or she has completed a series of training requirements, then passed a number of rigorous tests. Physicians who have not yet passed the certifying exam may be classified as *Board Eligible.*

Another factor is how much experience the physician you are considering has in treating your type of cancer. Remember, there are more than one hundred kinds of cancer. These, and their treatments, vary significantly. Still another important factor is to size up the comfort level you feel with the doctor at your initial meeting. However, remember that initial impressions do not always tell the entire story.

That was Cliff's experience. His initial contact with Dr. Horace Short, whom Cliff considered to be well-named because of his diminutive size, actually seemed to produce a level of hostility—particularly when Cliff brought up the subject of his personal faith. However, Cliff decided to give Dr. Short the benefit of the doubt, especially when he talked things over later with Dr. Handley, with whom he had a long-standing relationship. During the course of Cliff's treatment, that decision proved to be a good one. Cliff came to the conclusion that, although at times he had a strange way of showing it, Dr. Short did have a great deal of concern for his patients. Furthermore, he seemed to specialize in open communication, a fact Cliff appreciated greatly during the course of his treatment. And he was extremely skilled and knowledgeable in the treatment of Cliff's kind of cancer.

It is important to remember that, no matter how competent the physician you choose, you are ultimately your own patient advocate. You need to remain personally involved in the treatment process. And though it is important for your physician to include you in the many decisions to be made during the course of your care, you should take the initiative to exercise your right to accept or refuse any test or treatment suggested. Requesting a second or even a third opinion from another qualified medical professional is both appropriate and wise.

So be sure to be diligent to stay on top of all your checkups, appointments, and treatments. If you have more than one physician, make sure you see that each doctor who treats you is aware of what the other doctors are doing. Most important, don't hesitate to ask questions. A good physician welcomes healthy, honest questions and provides candid, competent answers to the best of his or her ability.

Preparing for Treatment

Before employing one or more of the three basic weapons—surgery, chemotherapy, or radiotherapy—the medical team will want to make sure of the specific classification (or grade) of cancer, its stage, and the degree of spread, or metastasis, if any (see chapter 2). As Cliff, Tom, Candy, Jessica, and other cancer patients have discovered, even the diagnosis of cancer can produce a great deal of discomfort. The process often begins when a person becomes aware of the cancer warning signs publicized by the American Cancer Society:

• unusual bleeding or discharge
• a lump that doesn't go away
• a sore that doesn't heal within two weeks
• a change in bowel or bladder habits
• persistent hoarseness or cough
• indigestion or difficulty in swallowing
• changes in a wart or a mole

Any of these indicators, or a persistent weight loss like Cliff experienced, should prompt a person to get an immediate checkup. Early diagnosis and prompt treatment is critical in successfully fighting cancer.

Numerous diagnostic tools are available to today's medical profession. Some are by nature noninvasive, such as the CAT scan, MRI, or ultrasound. Others involve injecting barium or some form of dye, then utilizing X rays to highlight internal features that otherwise could not be seen. Similar dyes can be injected into the kidney, bladder, and ureter.

Other procedures allow for the examination of tissue by a pathologist—for example, the Pap smear is a common tool used to check for the presence of cervical cancer in women. A standard hemoccult provides a test for the presence of blood in the stool—a possible indicator of colorectal cancer.

The primary goal of cancer treatment is to get rid of all the cancer cells in the patient's body.

Other diagnostic tools, such as the laparoscope, bronchoscope, endscope, or sigmoidoscope, allow the doctor to actually view the inside of different parts of the body through either natural openings or minute incisions. An eight-inch biopsy needle allows for tissues to be removed from a tumor in virtually any location within the body.

Frequently, blood tests can tell physicians a great deal about a person's condition—and about many kinds of cancer. Though these procedures may not be enjoyable, they constitute an essential part of the preparation for mobilizing the major weapons with which we treat cancer.

The Primary Goal of Treatment

The primary goal of cancer treatment is to get rid of all the cancer cells in the patient's body. There are basically two approaches to achieving this goal and four primary means. One approach is simply to cut away the cancerous tissue—the objective of surgery. The second is to kill the cancer cells in the body—the goal of radiotherapy, chemotherapy, and immuno-therapy.

The most common approach involves a combination of these treatments. The specific choices for any patient depend upon the precise diagnosis, the stage of the cancer involved, and the general health of the patient diagnosed with cancer. Once the diagnosis has been made, the cancer graded, and the stage of the tumor identified, the medical team can evaluate all the treatment options and come up with the most effective combination. In Cliff's case, Dr. Short recommended immediate surgery, to be followed by both radiation therapy and chemotherapy to kill any remaining cancer cells left in the body.

Cliff had been informed by Dr. Short and by Dr. Ventura, the surgical specialist, that the two of them recommended immediate surgery to remove the tumor. After raising a number of questions, Cliff and Gloria agreed. Their questions included expectations regarding what the surgery would accomplish, what the doctors would do during the operation, the risks of the surgery itself balanced against the risks of not having the surgery, the length of stay in the hospital, how long before Cliff could resume working, and even cost and insurance coverage.

Dr. Ventura noted that Cliff had not thought to ask about pain or pain control and suggested that this is fairly common of prospective surgical patients, since most preferred not to think of the prospect of pain. Then he outlined his plans for the surgical procedure. He also explained about the maze of machines and tubes that would be present and the professional staff members who would be working during the surgery.

"It's all high tech," Dr. Ventura explained. "We do things today we wouldn't have even considered a few years ago—we can take out a lung or amputate part of the liver—and we have machines that give us a constant monitor on the status of the patient, including blood pressure, the condition of the blood, heart waves, brain waves, lung pressure. In other words, you'll be in a pretty safe environment."

After voicing their questions and interacting over the proposed follow-up treatments with radiation and chemo, Cliff and Gloria finally voiced their agreement. "Let's get it underway," Cliff said. "Where do I sign?" Dr. Ventura's nurse brought in consent forms and things began to move ahead.

Cliff would check into the hospital after several days on a clear liquid diet and take numerous laxatives and enemas until his colon was completely clean in order to reduce the danger of infection. The day Cliff checked into the hospital, both his physicians reviewed his medical history carefully, going over the results of his lab tests. Dr. Ventura ordered a mild medication to help Cliff sleep.

Early the following morning, Gloria and Cliff's pastor, Frank, arrived just as the sun's rays were breaking over the hill behind the hospital. They entered Cliff's room just after the nurse had given Cliff his pre-op medication. Pastor Frank read several verses from Psalm 91 about God's watchcare over His children to encourage both Cliff and Gloria, then led in prayer, asking for God's hand of wisdom on the surgical team and for protection and strength for Cliff, as well as success in the surgery's mission of getting all the cancer. Cliff's "Amen" echoed that of Pastor Frank. He squeezed Gloria's hand, then said quietly but firmly, "Well, time to go," as an orderly pushed a gurney into the room.

The orderly transferred Cliff to the gurney, covered him with a blanket, then wheeled him down the hallway, with Gloria and Pastor Frank walking alongside as far as the waiting room. Automatic doors opened and Cliff was taken into the staging area of the surgery suite. After a brief delay he was wheeled into the operating room itself, where he was greeted by the anesthesiologist. At this point the process of prepping for surgery began in earnest.

Good news: Cliff's liver
was free from cancer.

Within the surgical suite every possible precaution was taken to protect Cliff from infection. The entire surgical team was clothed in sterilized garments. Paper wraps covered their shoes and hair, and masks covered their mouths and noses. While one member of the team arranged an array of sterilized surgical instruments, a nurse swabbed Cliff's arm with an antiseptic, then carefully inserted a needle linked by a plastic tube to a bottle of liquid—an IV. As Cliff chatted with the anesthesiologist, another nurse inserted a catheter to keep Cliff's bladder empty during surgery. The anesthesiologist attached his drip to the IV, and before long Cliff drifted into unconsciousness.

At this point Dr. Short and Dr. Ventura entered the surgical suite, hands held out in front of them. The two men had been scrubbing their hands and forearms for several minutes with a powerful antiseptic soap. Cliff's abdomen had been carefully cleansed and the surgical field shaved to remove any hair that might harbor bacteria. Checking briefly with the anesthesiologist, Dr. Ventura called for a scalpel and the operation itself was underway.

With a quick incision, Dr. Ventura opened Cliff's abdomen, then identified and tied several blood vessels. The two physicians carefully examined the contents of Cliff's abdomen. They not only checked his entire colon, but also examined his liver, since colon cancer frequently spreads to the liver. Good news: Cliff's liver was free from cancer.

However, in the course of checking a series of nearby lymph nodes, Dr. Ventura pointed to one, then looked up at Dr. Short, his brow knit in a frown. "Looks like it's enlarged," Dr. Short observed, nodding agreement.

Dr. Ventura quickly removed the lymph node, handing it to a nurse to be taken to the pathologist for a frozen section to quickly determine the possible presence of cancer cells. Other bits of tissue were also carefully removed, labeled, and given to the pathologist.

Within minutes, the report from the pathology lab came back. The cells from the enlarged lymph node were malignant. The other samples, however, indicated that the cancer was confined to the tumor in Cliff's transverse colon and the nearby enlarged lymph node.

Working rapidly, Dr. Ventura removed just under two feet of the colon, plus a portion of the mesentery, an apron of fat, blood vessels, and lymph nodes. The surgeon's work was done with quick but gentle movements in order to avoid dislodging cancer cells into the bloodstream where they might metastasize to other parts of Cliff's body. Large nearby veins were isolated, then tied off, as was one of the three major arteries supplying blood to the colon. Whereas some colon surgeries result in a colostomy, or artificial opening, either temporary or permanent, in the abdominal wall to which a small bag is attached to handle the colon's output, this was not necessary in Cliff's case.

The anesthesiologist had been carefully observing the machines that registered Cliff's pulse rate, breathing, blood pressure, and blood content, watching for any danger signs. Before long, Dr. Ventura completed the task of cutting away the tissue from well above and below the tumor. He then used a heavy suture to splice the two ends of the bowel back together. Almost two hours had gone by since the surgery began.

Dr. Ventura called for a sponge count—a procedure taken seriously by every surgical team. As soon as the circulating nurse called out that the sponge count was correct, Dr. Ventura began closing Cliff's surgical incision, confident that no sponges had been inadvertently left inside. Before long Cliff was wheeled into the recovery room, where his vital signs were carefully monitored and specially trained nurses helped him back to consciousness.

Back in the nearby waiting room, Gloria and Pastor Frank had been waiting, sipping from Styrofoam cups of coffee, praying together, and discussing a variety of topics. Since their church has a relatively small number of members, and because of his close relationship with Cliff and Gloria, Frank decided to wait with Gloria until the surgeon's return with word about the operation.

The Postoperative Report

Calling Gloria's name, Dr. Ventura and Dr. Short invited her to step into a private room just outside the surgical waiting area. She motioned for Pastor Frank to follow. The physicians' report was concise, as optimistic as possible, but candid. "The surgery went well. We expect a full recovery. We were able to get the tumor out without any difficulty. There was no cancer in the liver, and we were able to resect the bowel without the need for a colostomy. Our biggest concern is that one lymph node tested positive, so we need to monitor Cliff's situation carefully."

Within a couple of hours, Cliff was returned to his hospital bed. He was still quite groggy and a bit irritable—normal responses after major surgery. Cliff's nurse encouraged him to take a few sips of water—most of his nutrition came from the

IV, which also maintained a balance in the electrolytes in his blood. Before long the nurse returned to the room, urging Cliff to take deep breaths; a bit later, he was encouraged to hang his feet over the edge of the bed. Within hours he would be sitting up, and by the next day, he would actually be taking steps.

In recent years, surgeons have discovered that the former common practice of keeping surgery patients immobilized for days actually hindered the healing process. A carefully monitored pattern of increasing exercise—even when the patient is reluctant—can provide the key to a quicker recovery from the trauma of surgery.

Before long Cliff had taken sips of water, then clear liquids, including apple juice and cola. The first evening he didn't feel well, but by the next day he told Dr. Short and Dr. Ventura the line for which he would soon become noted among his friends: "You guys left me with a semicolon."

As soon as Cliff's stitches were removed, Dr. Short again reviewed his current status and prognosis for the future. Cliff was made completely aware that the cancer had metastasized into nearby lymph node tissue. The official diagnosis, confirmed by the pathologist, was an adenocarcinoma of the sigmoid colon.

The oncologist was candid to the point of bluntness. "To be honest, Cliff, adenocarcinoma sometimes doesn't respond very well to either radiation or chemo. But I think we were able to catch this pretty early. I'll be honest. I really think you should have a round of radiation, followed up by chemo."

---

*There are a number of benefits
to radiation therapy.*

"How do you see my chances now, Doc? Level with me."

"When I first entered medical practice twenty years ago, one of my first patients had almost the identical cancer, about the same size and same place, and he's still alive and well today. But to be candid, the statistics are just about even on whether you will or will not have a recurrence.

"I think the best way to go is a round of radiation to focus on the area near where we removed the tumor—especially some of the lymph nodes that were right next to the one we took out that was malignant. Then I think chemo can help take care of any cancer cells that may have spread through your bloodstream."

Later that evening Cliff reviewed his conversation with Dr. Short with Gloria and his oldest son, a seventeen-year-old who had expressed an interest in studying medicine. "Doc thinks I need a few sessions with the cobalt bomb," Cliff reported. Candidly he expressed a degree of fear regarding the radiation— primarily of the side effects. Cliff, Gloria, and their son expressed agreement about the risks, while encouraging Cliff to go ahead with the radiation. After the three of them prayed together, Cliff nodded. "I think it's the thing to do."

Radiation Therapy

The point of radiotherapy is to destroy cancer cells using intense doses of high-energy radiation under careful control. The chances of unpleasant side effects are high—intense nausea or vomiting, feelings of exhaustion, hair loss, and others.

Radiation can be used to shrink tumors prior to surgery or, as in Cliff's case, to clean up cancer cells that may be left in an area following surgery. Sometimes during surgery *seeds* of radiation are implanted in or near an area of surgery—sometimes temporarily, occasionally permanently.

Sometimes a radioactive material is given by injection, or even orally. However, the most common form of radiation treatment is external—using a machine to focus a high-energy beam on a precise location known to be malignant. In recent years, radiotherapy has improved to the point that, in some cases, lower doses of radiation are needed, and there is less damage to nearby tissue and fewer side effects.

There are a number of benefits to radiation therapy. It usually takes a shorter amount of time than chemotherapy, and it can be used on people who are not strong enough for surgery. Radiotherapy can reach areas that perhaps cannot be reached with surgery, and it may leave less radical physical changes than with some surgery, such as a mastectomy. Some of the newest developments in radiation therapy, including proton therapy, can actually focus millions of volts of radiation precisely on the site of a tumor without affecting nearby healthy tissue. Radiation is the treatment of choice for such malignancies as Hodgkin's disease and lymphoma.

Since Dr. Short was an oncologist who had specialized in radiotherapy, he would supervise Cliff's radiation treatments. As Dr. Short prepared for Cliff to begin the radiation therapy, additional CAT scans were ordered to determine with pinpoint accuracy where the radiation beams would be focused.

Dr. Short explained to Cliff in even greater detail than before the possibility of side effects, then scheduled a series of five, five-day treatments. He warned Cliff that this would be an ordeal but added that successful completion of the course of radiation treatment could be the key to Cliff's survival.

Cliff's treatments were given on an outpatient basis in the nuclear medicine department of the same hospital where his surgery was performed. During the final visit to Dr. Short's office prior to beginning the radiation treatment, the oncologist carefully located and marked on Cliff's abdomen the location, known as the *treatment port*, with indelible ink. This was the precise spot at which the radiation would be aimed during each of the treatments. The point of scheduling radiation treatments over a course of time is to prevent, as much as possible, any harm to nearby healthy tissues.

Cliff was just beginning to regain his health from the surgery, so Gloria offered to drive him for the treatments. Each visit to the hospital took approximately an hour, sometimes more—although the actual time Cliff spent each treatment under the "cobalt bomb" was less than a minute.

Dressed only in a hospital gown, Cliff was placed on the treatment table. Portions of his body were covered with lead shielding, and the technician carefully positioned the radiation machine over the treatment port.

"Will this hurt?" Cliff asked as he prepared for the initial session. It was a question he hadn't thought to raise with Dr. Short.

"Not a bit," the technician responded, grinning. "It will probably hurt me worse than it does you. Hold real still now."

The technician closed a heavy door, and Cliff was left alone on the table, awaiting the radiation. In a moment he heard a sound like a distant jet engine revving faster, but he didn't feel a thing. After a minute the sound stopped, and the technician returned to the room, joking with Cliff and removing the lead shields.

Soon Cliff became used to the routine of the treatments. Initially he didn't feel nauseated, but within a week he noted a loss of appetite—something he had just begun to regain following the surgery. He also reported feeling nauseated and experiencing some vomiting and diarrhea.

Dr. Short assured Cliff that these were fairly normal symptoms, particularly with radiation to the abdomen. He urged Cliff to continue eating, even when he didn't feel hungry, and suggested yogurt, cottage cheese, and fruit.

Cliff replied, "I'm basically a meat and potatoes guy, Doc."

"Not anymore, Cliff. Not anymore."

Cliff also reported feeling quite a bit of fatigue during the third week of his radiation therapy. "I don't want to be a complainer, Doc," he told Dr. Short, "but I really need to get my energy back."

"Better to lose your energy now and keep yourself alive," Dr. Short responded with characteristic straightforwardness. "Just a couple of weeks to go now. You're big on the Bible. Doesn't it talk about things passing away?"

Some people tolerate chemo with very few side effects. For others, it's pretty tough.

Forcing a tired smile, Cliff nodded. "OK, Doc. I'll hang in there. I guess I'm just expecting more of myself than I have to give right now."

"That's common, Cliff. You need to cut yourself some slack. After all, the main thing for you right now is to get this part of your treatment over with. Then we'll move on to chemo. Hopefully by the time that's done, we'll have your cancer licked."

Chemical Therapy

As the term itself suggests, chemotherapy is the use of chemicals to treat a disease. Technically, any use of chemical medicines—pain killers, antibiotics, blood pressure medication—could be called chemotherapy. In the field of cancer treatment, however, the term *chemotherapy* refers to the use of chemicals that kill cancer cells.

To many people the term itself is extremely frightening. Some individuals have the idea that chemotherapy is a last resort, prescribed only when things are hopeless. As Dr. Short was quick to assure Cliff, that isn't the case at all. The well-meaning individual who had suggested to Cliff that chemotherapy would only be used as a last resort was misguided.

"Let me also caution you not to make the intensity of the side effects a gauge of the success of the chemotherapy," Dr. Short continued. "The reason I mention this is that some people think that chemo doesn't work unless it makes you terribly sick. To be candid, it depends on both the chemical used and the individual. Some people tolerate chemo with very few side effects. For others, it's pretty tough. But you generally can expect some pretty unpleasant side effects. That's the biggest drawback to chemo. The main reason is—and I'll be blunt about it—we're poisoning you to help kill any leftover cancer: those tiny cells that may have been dislodged during your surgery and floated through your body to lodge in some remote spot—perhaps your lungs or pancreas."

Although he didn't know it, Dr. Short's statement would prove to be prophetic. After several years of freedom from colon cancer, Cliff would one day be diagnosed with cancer of the pancreas. Fighting cancer would continue to be a major part of his life.

"Cliff," Dr. Short continued, "I want to warn you. Sometimes the side effects are so bad that patients decide to give up on the program—quit right in the middle of the treatment. I've seen it happen too many times. So I want to encourage you not to quit."

"I'm not a quitter, Doc," Cliff replied. "I'm sure I don't have any idea how bad this may be—but I'll hang in there."

It didn't take long before Cliff found out exactly what Dr. Short meant. Unfortunately, there are still some oncologists who minimize the side effects of chemotherapy with comments like, "Oh, you may feel a little nauseous at times." We feel it is most appropriate for doctors to be honest yet compassionate in discussing possible side effects of chemo with their patients. The biblical principle is always to speak "the truth in love"

(Ephesians 4:15). Although he did not profess to be a Christian, Dr. Short did choose to follow Paul's recommended approach to communication. He told Cliff the truth, and did so lovingly, if at times a bit brusquely.

For Cliff, as for many others, chemotherapy proved both good and bad. Good in that it helped destroy cancer—for five years, he was cancer free. Bad in that it left him intensely nauseated, sometimes so violently ill that he actually found himself wishing he could die rather than throw up anymore.

What little appetite he had left following the radiation therapy totally disappeared once the chemotherapy began. Dr. Short prescribed antinausea medication, but it only left Cliff feeling barely alive. There were intestinal cramps and diarrhea —this in an intestine just recovering from the traumatic effects of surgery.

Before long, Cliff noticed his hair falling out in great clumps each time he combed it. Within days, his entire shock of thick, sandy hair had disappeared. Managing a weak smile he told his young son, "I always wanted to play basketball like Kareem Abdul-Jabbar, or Charles Barkley. Now at least I have the look!" While Gloria suggested a wig, Dr. Short recommended a cap—the suggestion Cliff followed, although he seemed to have a hard time getting used to wearing a cap indoors.

Unlike radiation therapy, which usually takes place over a brief span measured generally in weeks, Cliff's chemotherapy lasted nearly six months. During the third month Cliff raised a common question, "Why do I need to continue with this chemo anyway? It's just making my life miserable. Why not just give me another quick round of radiation therapy? After all, a few more blasts from the cobalt bomb would sure be better than spending half my life hanging over the toilet bowl, turning my insides out."

"I'm sure you rate me somewhere between Simon Legree and Attila the Hun for prescribing what seems like torture," Dr. Short replied curtly. "But I'll be honest with you, Cliff. There's one big advantage to chemotherapy. It's systemic. In other words, when we use chemo we're treating the entire system—your whole body. When we operated on you, Dr. Ventura was very careful to ensure that we did as little dislodging as possible. But there's absolutely no way we can be sure that either before or during surgery some cancer cells didn't slip into the bloodstream. Chemotherapy has the best chance of killing cancer cells anywhere in your body."

"Why does it have to take so long?" asked Gloria, who had accompanied Cliff for the visit.

"First order kinetics," Dr. Short shot back, smiling as he noted the puzzled look on both Cliff's and Gloria's faces. "That means we keep killing the cancer cells in your body at a relatively constant rate. Say for example, one round of drugs kills 75 percent of the cancer cells in your body. The next round kills 75 percent of the remaining 25 percent. And the next round, 75 percent of what's left then. Pretty soon we get the number of cancer cells down to a level your own immune system can handle. That's why I plan to utilize one more strategy—something called immunotherapy."

Biological Therapy

"A relatively new, somewhat experimental approach to treating cancer, biological therapy, or immunotherapy, involves utilizing new medications designed to boost the body's immune system to fight cancer," Dr. Short explained. "After all, millions of years of evolution have produced a better cancer fighting system than medicine could ever come up with—and chemicals like interferon and CSFs are just a means we can use to support that system."

Cliff smiled at Dr. Short's comment. "Or it may be that a wise Creator simply designed a system that works better than medicine—that seems to be a pretty plausible explanation, wouldn't you think?" Cliff held up his wristwatch. "I'm wearing a Timex, and I couldn't help noticing that you're wearing a Rolex. But neither of us would suggest that our timepieces simply evolved over millions of years. Someone more intelligent than the intelligence of the watch itself had to design the watch."

"Not to change the subject," Dr. Short huffed, "but I guess I ought to explain CSFs to you. You're probably wondering what that meant. They're called *colony stimulating factors* that will stimulate the body's immune system—the major defense against foreign substances. It's the main protection against infection by bacteria, as well as the primary natural defense against cancer. CSFs stimulate the production of cells such as the T-cells that could recognize a cancer cell as foreign and attack it. Another approach is to use what we call TNFs—tumor necrosis factors—to actually enhance the capability of the body to kill tumor cells.

"In fact, Cliff, it's actually thought that most people develop cancers on an almost ongoing basis through life, but the immune system eliminates them. This has been proven, for example, with some of the research done into T-cell leukemia, a cancer of the white blood cells. The National Cancer Institute has isolated a virus they called HTLV-1, or human T-lymphocyte leukemia virus, which actually set the stage for some of the research into the HIV virus. The point is, this research didn't prove that all cancer was caused by viruses. But it did prove that at least in some cases—this one in particular—a virus was the culprit. Cervical cancer, which is pretty common in premenopausal women, has been linked with a virus called HPV—human papilloma virus—which is also connected with some sexually transmitted diseases.

"I'm not a Christian, mind you, but I do think Christian moral standards could actually cut down on the risk of cancer. For example, if women have multiple sexual partners, the risk of developing cervical cancer increases pretty significantly. My point is, there is a pretty clear-cut link between viruses and cancer. And the biological response of the body can be modified by drugs like interferon, interleukin, and other agents. Ideally, if we could *completely* manipulate your immune system, we could eliminate the need for chemotherapy. We'd just have your immune system selectively kill all the cancer cells without damaging normal tissues."

"You've lost me, Doc—at least I think you have," Cliff jumped in. "What are interferons? Cells that interfere with something?"

Another smile spread across Dr. Short's face. "Sorry. Interferons and interleukins are actually groups of proteins produced by cells in the immune system. They're pretty complex. But the big benefit is, these are naturally occurring anticancer substances. There's been a lot of work in genetic engineering. For example, we can fuse a lymphocyte—which produces an antibody specifically for a cancer cell—inside a cell from some other mammal, then inject these cells called monoclonal antibodies into the bloodstream. They travel through the bloodstream like a military search party until they encounter a tumor cell, then attach themselves to it. If we attach a radioactive molecule—sort of a "label" to the antibody—we can actually trace the monoclonal antibodies by concentration and pinpoint isolated locations of tumor cells that we couldn't otherwise find. We can also attach some of the newer chemotherapy drugs— we call them oncotoxins—to these antibodies, and they will actually kill the tumor cells. There's a lot of work left to be done in this area, but immunotherapy has a great future, especially when it's used in combination with chemo."

In Cliff's case, the chemicals for his treatment were taken in two forms: a monthly injection, and a daily sequence of pills for three weeks out of every month. Both the injections and the pills worsened Cliff's nausea, and he was given regular blood tests to determine whether either his red or white cell count had dropped too low.

Treatment Completed

Following six months of chemotherapy, Cliff was finally told that his treatments were over. "You've been a good patient, Cliff. I've appreciated your persistence and your cheerfulness despite the negative circumstances. And I'll admit, in your case what I've seen in terms of faith has been mighty impressive also. I'm glad you've done well."

As Cliff concluded his visit with Dr. Short, he said, "Doc, I'd like to thank you for everything you've done for me. You, Dr. Ventura, and Dr. Handley who first suspected I had cancer— you guys have played a big part in my treatment. But I'm not cured yet, am I?"

The chances for Cliff's cure looked good, but Dr. Short refused to pronounce him cured."No, Cliff, not yet. We'll not call you *cured* until there's been no detectable evidence of cancer for at least five years. At that point, we would consider you to have the same life expectancy as if you never had cancer. So take care of yourself. Keep abreast of some of the developments in cancer research—the clinical trials. And keep coming back for those checkups—every three months, whether you think you need them or not."

"OK, Doc. I'll see you in ninety days. And I'm convinced that with God on my side and with you and the rest of my treatment team, we'll be able to handle whatever comes our way."

Dr. Short didn't say anything for a moment. Cliff noticed him swallow twice. "Maybe sometime soon I can take you to lunch," Cliff said. "You know, outside the medical arena. Just to get together and visit."

Dr. Short frowned, his dark eyebrows bunching together. "Cliff, I make it a point never to fraternize with my patients outside the office." Then he continued with a twinkle in his eye, "But, I'm not sure that's a policy I need to worry about following. Sure, let's get together for lunch sometime."

That evening as Cliff and Gloria celebrated a conclusion of his treatment at their favorite seafood restaurant, Cliff commented, "Who knows? Maybe I'll have a chance to tell that oncologist of mine about God's treatment for a problem that's even more fatal than cancer."

9

ENCOURAGING THE CANCER PATIENT'S FAMILY

Even though less than a year had passed since Shannon lost her husband Jim to pancreatic cancer, she hadn't lost her sense of humor. Laughter frequently punctuated the conversation as she shared the story of a two-year battle against a form of disease that cancer expert Dr. Mark Renneker calls "among the most deadly and frightening of all cancers; few survive and the incidence is increasing."[1] But there were also times when grief, and even anger, surfaced during the discussion—grief over her loss, and anger over the pain and suffering Jim's cancer had caused them both.

Approximately 26,000 cases of pancreatic cancer are diagnosed each year in the United States—representing a 25 percent increase since the 1950s. No single cause has been isolated, although possible culprits include tobacco smoke, coffee, and alcohol. Remembering something she once heard, Shannon said, "Mormons and Seventh Day Adventists have extremely low rates of pancreatic cancer, so tobacco, alcohol, and caffeine may be part of the risk factor."

Dr. Jim Mahoney had served as a pastor and an evangelist for many years. He participated in the founding of Rapha Treatment Centers and served as one of its first therapists. He never used alcohol or tobacco. But he did have another risk factor. "Soda and junk food. He was just a junk food junkie," Shannon recalled. "When we were working together on the first Rapha unit in Galveston, Jim knew everywhere and at what time the donuts would come out hot. He loved any kind of junk food. And he seldom drank water. Soft drinks, yes. Water, no. He would drink just a little coffee, and even less water. He would take just a few sips from a soft drink, then set it aside. After his cancer diagnosis, when we discovered he had diabetes, it was because he drank two sodas in a row one day that tipped us off that something was wrong."

But diabetes didn't develop until well into "Doc" Mahoney's battle with cancer—a battle shared every step of the way by his energetic young bride of six years. And as Shannon recounted the story of how they fought the disease together, one factor surfaced over and over: the encouragement and support they gave each other, plus the encouragement of a circle of friends and family members, played a key role in sustaining Jim and Shannon during those dark, difficult days.

Doc—a Skilled Encourager

That Dr. Jim Mahoney would receive support and encouragement during his fight with cancer wasn't surprising. After all, Shannon was not the only one who remembered him as being "the epitome of God's unconditional love and acceptance for people." A regular participant on the "Life Perspectives" radio call-in ministry during its early days, Doc delighted in sharing insight and encouragement with hurting people. He was a skilled and gifted encourager who genuinely cared for others.

Doc had worked closely with Rapha founder and president Robert McGee in developing the material that would become the basis for Robert's best-selling book *The Search for Significance,* and he took special delight in having crafted a technique for applying biblical principles and scriptural truths to overcome false beliefs and destructive emotions—a process that came to be called "the trip in." Laughing one day during a break in a live call-in radio program, Doc responded to a question about "the trip in."

"I had always heard that hippies and people involved in drugs talk about 'tripping out.' So when Robert and I first started thinking about this concept, we felt the best thing to call it was 'the trip in.' After all, it was designed to let individuals look inside themselves, find out where false beliefs were affecting their emotions and behaviors, and change those false beliefs based on biblical truths such as redemption, reconciliation, and propitiation. It was a way to get Bible doctrine into personal experience."

More than one of his colleagues referred to Jim's role at Rapha during those days as "the heart of the organization." According to Shannon, that characterization was right on target. "He had such a deep heart and longing for people. He was willing and able to take the most difficult patients" who entered the Christian treatment program at Rapha—even those other therapists might have been tempted to give up on. In his conference ministry as well as on the radio, Jim Mahoney would address such practical topics as anger, loneliness, and depression with compassion and spiritual wisdom.

One of Doc's favorite responsibilities with Rapha involved *Stress In Ministry* conferences designed to provide encouragement for hurting pastors. The heartfelt desire to help stressed-out ministers and ministers' wives was shared by Jim and Shannon alike. As he once put it, "Nobody outside the ministry fully understands what men in ministry or their wives have to go through. I'm just glad we can help them process some of their pain and encourage them to keep on without giving up." From Shannon's perspective, "I don't think there was anything any closer to Jim's heart than *Stress In Ministry.*"

"The doctors couldn't explain the constant, chronic pain."

Just slightly on the stocky side of slim, Jim had piercing blue eyes, an engaging smile, and thinning, sandy hair. "He was a great Houston Oilers football fan," Shannon remembered. "I could always spot him in the crowd at Oiler games whenever I came back to my seat. I'd tease him about his bald spot, because that's how I would pick him out of the crowd." Doc never minded being teased, and he didn't mind teasing others either.

Shannon first met Doc Mahoney one night when he filled the pulpit at the church she was attending near Houston. "The pastor had died unexpectedly. It was the night we were dedicating our new family center." From that first meeting a friendship developed that lasted several years and included a time when both worked on one of the earliest Rapha units. Before long, to the delight of their colleagues, the friendship had blossomed into a romance, which ultimately ripened into matrimony.

For three years following their marriage, things were blissful in every way. Then slowly but surely, Shannon began to notice that Doc was experiencing a lot of physical discomfort. Stomach and digestive problems became increasingly frequent. "He had had stomach troubles off and on ever since I knew him. But things were getting noticeably worse. So Doc and I decided it was time for the two of us to go in and get physicals—after all, we were both well overdue. We also decided to work together to start eating proper foods and exercising regularly."

Doc Got Worse and Worse

Doc and Shannon started being careful to eat correctly and exercise, and Doc made it a point to follow his physician's instructions to "drink lots of water"—even though he hated drinking water. But Doc's pain became worse and worse.

Since Doc was traveling a great deal, speaking on behalf of Rapha and ministering in churches across the country, both he and Shannon felt that his pain was caused by the strain of traveling and the difficulty of eating correctly that resulted from his heavy schedule. A visit to an internist resulted in a referral to a gastrointestinal specialist—"a GI guy"—who concluded that Doc's problem was irritable bowel syndrome. "I went to the library," Shannon recalled. "Checked out all the books I could find on the subject—brought them home. Doc and I poured over them. We concluded the diagnosis must be right. It certainly sounded like his symptoms. However, the books said that irritable bowel pain was more intermittent. His pain had become chronic."

On a Friday morning during the summer of 1990, Doc and Shannon found out what they were *really* up against. The pain had worsened, and Shannon recalled that "Jim just couldn't sit up. He couldn't lie down. We had no explanation for why the pain kept getting worse, even though he was following the doctor's instructions about diet and drinking water. The doctors couldn't explain the constant, chronic pain, even with an inflamed, irritable bowel."

Shannon recalled learning later that such pain was unusual for pancreatic cancer. "We found out that his tumor was located right next to the major nerve in the pancreas. That was actually a help in our getting the right treatment promptly for Jim." The location of the pancreas—a thin, six-inch-long gland straddling the stomach and intestines—plus the presence of just one primary nerve, makes finding and diagnosing pancreatic cancer in time for effective treatment an extreme rarity. "We discovered that cancer of the pancreas has the distinction of being the most deadly of all major cancers. Of every one hundred people who get it, ninety will be dead within a year. And the remaining ten almost certainly will die within five years. The problem is, it's so hard to diagnose. Because of Jim's pain, which resulted from a tiny tumor close to the major nerve in the pancreas, his cancer was diagnosed more quickly than usual."

"It was the week of the Fourth of July—a hot, humid time in Houston, as summertime so frequently is. We went back to the internist. We were his last appointment of the day. Because of Jim's intense pain, he curled up in a ball on the examining table. The doctor immediately said, 'We'll have to put you in the hospital and run some more tests. There seems to be more to this than just irritable bowel.'" That day Jim checked into the hospital and began undergoing a series of diagnostic procedures on his gastrointestinal tract.

Doc's Supportive Friends

Several close friends rallied around Jim and Shannon to provide encouragement and support. "Patty, a good friend of mine, had lost her husband to lymphoma a few years before. When she remarried, it was to an oncologist, Dr. Roger Rodgers. We never had trouble remembering his name." Shannon chuckled.

"Because of our friendship with Patty, she asked Roger to take a look at Jim's situation. At that point we hadn't even considered the possibility of cancer. Roger actually made the discovery. I recall him asking Jim's doctors to run one more test, an MRI. They had already done a CAT scan, which didn't show anything. And normally a CAT scan is the best diagnostic tool to find pancreatic cancer. But nothing showed on Jim's CAT scan."

The next day, July Fourth, they ran the MRI. The initial results again seemed to indicate all clear. At this point the network of friends expanded. "I remember Delvin Kendricks coming that day. From then on, he was with us almost daily— loving, encouraging, supporting us. Ron Johnson, a young man who thought of Jim as a father or a mentor, also came that day."

Later that afternoon, Shannon recalled that Delvin, Ron, and Jim's internist were all in Jim's hospital room together. "I walked into that room, and Jim was sitting up in bed crying." Dropping everything, Shannon rushed to her husband's bedside to embrace him.

"We didn't understand it. The doctor had actually suggested that Jim might need psychiatric care to handle the pain more effectively, since he had obviously become depressed. Now, depression is a symptom of pancreatic cancer. Plus, we had already realized that Jim's pain was different—more steady and intense than what would be expected from irritable bowel. But until the diagnosis of pancreatic cancer, we were confused and devastated. The doctor told us pain management was an option but that this pain was something Jim would just have to live with."

About 9:00 the following morning, Shannon and Jim were talking over their options with their friends. "We were not opposed to psychiatric care; after all, we were both part of a team that delivered Christian-based psychiatric care to other people. So if that's what we had to do, that's what we would do."

Still unsure of anything but the reality of Jim's pain and the difficulty of dealing with it, the Mahoneys and their two friends began to discuss preparations for going home. "A few hours later Ron Johnson was still in the room with us. Another of the gastrointestinal doctors came in to tell us that plans had changed. They would be keeping Jim for additional tests."

Short—just over five feet—Dr. Bali, a native of India, explained. "We've looked things over carefully. We believe there is something else here. We think we've spotted something on the MRI. But we can't find out any more unless we run some additional tests."

Shannon recalled Dr. Bali mentioning several possibilities. "Two words he used stuck out to me—*tumor* and *pancreas*. And that's exactly what it turned out to be." When she heard the word *tumor,* Shannon came out of her chair. "It really hit me."

> *It is crucial for the cancer patient and the family to have a supportive circle of family and friends.*

Shannon recalled becoming increasingly more upset after the doctor's brief visit had raised the possibility that what Jim had was cancer. "It was just Providence that Ron was there right at that point. He was a nurse—he and Jim had worked together in a psychiatric care program even prior to Rapha, treating substance abuse patients. He also had worked with Jim in the early days of Rapha as one of our charge nurses."

According to Shannon, Ron's calm demeanor and careful explanation helped stabilize what was a volatile experience. "Wait, Shannon. This could explain it. This could explain Jim's pain. After all, pancreatitis produces steady, intense pain. Maybe that's Jim's problem."

Practical Encouragement

When cancer comes into a person's life, it is crucial for the cancer patient and the family to have a supportive circle of family and friends. As Doc and Shannon discovered (and as Cliff and his wife, Candy and her husband, and Jessica and her parents found out), the entire family goes through the treatment process together. Shannon agreed. "Both of us were put through the wringer. I desperately needed encouragement."

Having people who were there over the long haul made the difference, not only on that dark day when she learned that her husband was carrying a killer tumor in his body, but also during the difficult days and months that would lie ahead—including endless trips for therapy, sleepless nights, countless hours spent washing and rewashing clothes, and taking care of the routine chores that weigh so heavily. So what can be done to encourage the cancer patient *and* his or her family?

BE THERE

First, be there. Make contact. Follow the advice of the old telephone company commercial: "Reach out and touch someone." That seems so simple, so basic, that it almost goes without saying. Yet it needs to be said, then repeated over and over. Because when cancer comes, friends and family are often frightened into breaking off contact. After all, a disease like cancer reminds us of our own mortality.

As one close friend and work colleague of Jim's put it, "I didn't spend nearly as much time as I would have liked to with Doc. To be honest, I just couldn't handle it. I would stop by briefly, then stay away for weeks, even months. Then I would go by for another visit—a brief one."

We have seen this response time and again. Paralyzed by fear, potentially supportive family and friends stay away, making the battle against cancer harder. For some cancer patients and their families, there is an almost complete breakdown in the potential support system. For others, like Doc and Shannon, there are those who defy the trend and maintain support.

For Shannon Mahoney, having people who were there during those critical times made all the difference in the world. "You might say I was a professional at dealing with pain," said Shannon, a Rapha therapist who has dedicated her life to helping others deal with personal hurts. "But I needed people like Ron and Dr. Rodgers and Delvin. Then there was Annie. She was like a spiritual mom to me. She came consistently, time after time. And there was Kim, my roommate from college. She had come to the Lord after our college days, and it had produced a drastic change in her life. She really supported me. Prayed for Doc and me. Came and spent time."

What cancer patients and their families need most is a loving, reassuring presence—not a sermon, not deep theological insights, not even a collection of kind words, although kind words can certainly be appreciated. The initial and perhaps most important principle is simply to be there. Even a brief visit can be helpful—and sometimes brief is better than extended. But when there is a close relationship, when it is obvious the person needs someone there—stay, if at all possible. Change your schedule if necessary. Drop other things. Make arrangements to invest time. When family or close friends face the crisis of cancer, the way to spell love for them or their families is quite simply T-I-M-E. "I can't believe the amount of time Ron and Dr. Rodgers and Delvin and Annie and Kim and others spent with us," Shannon recalled. "I mean, they were *there* when we needed them."

Eye contact, appropriate physical contact, a warm handshake, a hand on a shoulder, a hug—all of these communicate the love and acceptance that people facing cancer or similar trials need. And all require being present.

The three friends who came to comfort Job during his time of sickness and loss provide a biblical example of how to be an encouragement and how not to be. Initially, Eliphaz, Bildad, and Zophar followed procedures that would work extremely well today. When they heard of his adversity, they came to where Job was (Job 2:11). They initiated this visit by setting an appointment to come together. Making such a commitment, letting the patient know that you plan to be there, can be an important source of encouragement. Keeping the commitment to come is of equal, or perhaps greater, importance. Job's three friends delivered on what they promised.

The three friends came with a twofold purpose: "to mourn with him and to comfort him" (v. 11). They apparently not only came to grieve with him according to the custom of the day, "lifting their voices and weeping, tearing their outer robes, and sprinkling dust on their heads toward heaven" (v. 12), they intended to share positive support with Job as well. They showed their support by sitting with Job for a period of seven days and seven nights without saying a word (v. 13). Here is the epitome of what encouraging friends can do. Sensing the pain of his grief, they simply waited. They were there for him. Bible teacher and counselor Gary Smalley has crafted a descriptive word picture to explain what that means. He calls it "being in your boat."

"Picture yourself alone in a boat in the middle of a lake in a storm," Gary told a caller one evening on "Life Perspectives" radio. "You're out there all by yourself. What do you need? Not a sermon. Not even a set of instructions for rowing the boat or cranking its motor. What I think you would appreciate most of all is somebody who would just be there with you in the boat."

That's the essence of encouragement—and the first step toward supporting both the cancer patient and his or her family.

However, Job's friends soon began to illustrate how *not* to comfort and encourage someone in intense physical or emotional pain. As soon as Job began to verbalize his grief, they launched into an extended dialogue developed around their self-professed theme that Job's suffering and sickness must be a direct result of some hidden sin: "Whoever perished being innocent, or where were the upright ever cut off?" (Job 4:7).

Shannon recalled that a few people during Jim's sickness, and even after he died, occasionally tended to preach at her. "I was told once or twice by people that I really should look for the good in this, and I heard Romans 8:28 quoted a time or two when I really wasn't ready to hear it. I needed time to grieve, to process my feelings, to feel my pain." What a well-put reminder for those of us who may be tempted to dump our spiritual platitudes on those who are still in the throes of their pain.

CALM FOCUS

Two additional principles we recommend to would-be encouragers are to communicate calm and focus on issues and options. Shannon recalled how their friend Ron epitomized communicating calm. "I was becoming more and more upset that Friday after the internist hinted at the possibility of a tumor. Later, Jim's primary physician came into the room, pulled up a chair, and said, 'I need to tell both of you straight out. Jim has cancer.' He explained that a needle biopsy had been scheduled for Monday, then left. Basically, he told us things were hopeless and we should just prepare to go home, manage the pain, and die. At that point, Jim and I were both just about as upset as two people could be. Believe me, Ron provided the calm in the middle of a major storm!"

For six months Jim had been growing progressively worse, his pain intensifying. Shannon and Jim had both suspected that something was terribly wrong—but they had no idea what. Now their worst fears—and more—were confirmed as the doctor explained that he believed the only alternative was to stabilize Jim and send him home. After the physicians' visits, Ron encouraged Shannon and Doc to ventilate their feelings and shared encouraging words of hope, despite the grim news the doctors had delivered.

In response to Ron's verbal encouragement, Jim and Shannon vowed to continue fighting. "Ron reminded us that now we had an enemy and a direction to head in fighting it—even though at the time we didn't realize just how fatal pancreatic cancer was considered to be."

There is a time for friends to say nothing. But there is also a time to let people know there are options.

Then, just a few minutes after Jim's primary doctor had unloaded the pancreatic cancer bombshell, their friend Dr. Roger Rodgers, the oncologist, arrived. Dr. Rodgers had provided the impetus for another review of the scans from Jim's MRI. In the process a tiny tumor was spotted, lodged in the pancreas. Shannon saw Dr. Rodgers's efforts as providential. "I believe God was really in it—most people only live six months or less after they discover they have pancreatic cancer. God gave us quite a bit longer than that—eighteen months to be precise—and I believe Dr. Rodgers's persistence played a key part."

Dr. Rodgers had spotted the tumor in a most unusual site. Usually pancreatic tumors are located at one end of the pancreas or the other—doctors refer to them as the head and the tail. By the time the tumor hits the nerve, where Jim's was growing, half the organ may have been taken over by the tumor. Jim's tumor was incredibly small, but Dr. Rodgers had spotted it right next to the nerve near the center of the pancreas.

FOCUS ON ISSUES AND OPTIONS

Dr. Rodgers provided a concrete example of another specific step friends and family members can take to communicate encouragement and support to cancer patients and their families—focus on issues and options. Trying to think clearly during the shock and pain that comes with a diagnosis of cancer, or even during extended treatment, is difficult at best. There is a time for friends to say nothing. But there also is a time to let people know there are options, to help them think through alternatives and decide on an action plan—or even to reevaluate a plan of action that isn't working very well.

From her experience in helping Rapha patients, as well as through the encouragement given her by Dr. Rodgers and others, Shannon has seen from both sides how this process works. "Dr. Rodgers is a genius—and his parents must have had quite a sense of humor, naming him Roger. I still remember how he gently but straightforwardly communicated the facts about Jim's cancer. He told us that for some people it's a matter of weeks, a few months at most. He also explained to us how the location of Jim's tumor caused the intense pain—that it wasn't that Jim lacked the willpower or the ability to cope. He let us know that depression was a major clinical symptom of pancreatic cancer."

Shannon feels that Dr. Rodgers's loving focus on issues helped spare her from bitterness, and Jim from unnecessary grief. "If we had left the hospital with the diagnosis of irritable bowel syndrome, or without what we learned about pancreatic cancer from Roger, I would have felt incredibly bitter and angry—and it would have been like a death sentence for Jim to think he just had some stomach pain he couldn't handle, rather than knowing what he was really up against."

From Shannon's perspective, Dr. Rodgers provided a source of both immediate encouragement and ongoing support, as a physician and as a friend. "Time after time he stopped to talk with Jim and me. He didn't snow us—he painted an accurate picture. He told us that if we'd had a choice, this would not have been the cancer we would have chosen. But he did let us know that there were options, options that extended beyond just giving up and going home to wait for Jim to die.

"Furthermore, he took it on himself to get the ball rolling on some of those options when we agreed to his recommendations. Because he and his wife, Patty, were our friends, he became involved personally even beyond the usual role of a physician. He also took care of many of the treatment things— like expediting the results from Jim's needle biopsy so the surgery and follow-up treatments could be scheduled as quickly as possible. Jim and I agreed that Roger was like a love gift from God to us. Even though he started off as an unofficial consultant and friend, I had to tell Jim's primary physician that we wanted Roger on the team—we felt that since he was an oncologist, he was best qualified to deal with what Jim had."

When Shannon faced the unpleasant task of communicating this to Jim's primary physician, Ron Johnson and Delvin Kendricks were there with her, illustrating yet another important principle of support. That principle might be explained as, *Whenever possible be present for crises, unpleasant confrontations, or other circumstances*. Extra support will be needed.

BE PRESENT AT CRISIS TIMES

It is easier to be a friend when things are going well. However, when life is falling apart for our friends, when they face a crisis such as cancer, which may remind us of our own mortality, or when they are in the midst of extremely unpleasant circumstances, our friendship will prove itself by our presence and support. Today, as in biblical times, crises are times in which true friendship is proven in the fires of adversity: "A friend loves at all times and a brother is born for adversity" (Proverbs 17:17). Rodger Rogers, Ron Johnson, and Delvin Kendricks provided this kind of support for Jim and Shannon.

Delvin Kendricks had every reason to want to help Doc and Shannon. After all, Doc had been there for him years earlier, when Delvin's son had taken his life. "Jim helped him through that tragedy," Shannon recalled, "so Delvin had just an incredible love for Jim. Delvin, Roger, and Ron were there that morning when I had to tell Jim's original doctor that what he had recommended was not going to be an option for us—we weren't going to just take pain medication, go home, and give up."

Rapha was another source of immediate encouragement. Rapha's CEO, Don Sapaugh, came to the hospital within hours of Jim's cancer diagnosis. "He wanted to assure us not to worry about finances or work schedule. He felt it was important for me to know that I was free to be there with Jim through the treatment process." Other Rapha colleagues, including Freddie and Daniel Gage, also arrived shortly after Don's visit. "Freddie was so supportive—he visited and phoned often—and I'm convinced that he eventually had just about the entire Southern

Baptist Convention praying for Jim. Later, when Jim was nearing death, Freddie was the one person who had the courage to
ask Jim what he wanted done at his funeral. Then, within hours
of Jim's death, he took me to make all the funeral arrangements."

A support group in which she had participated as a part
of the Rapha unit at Spring Branch Hospital in Houston provided still another source of significant support for Shannon. She
viewed it as one of Rapha's best support groups. Shannon
headed to the group meeting within hours of hearing Jim's diagnosis. En route, she decided to stop off at the library at the
University of Texas Medical Center. She opened one of the medical textbooks to the section on pancreatic cancer. "I just had to
shut it. It overwhelmed me when I read about the mortality rate
and everything associated with it. I just couldn't handle it. I'd
gone down to the library prepared to check out everything they
had and study up on it. But I just couldn't do it."

Feeling overwhelmed, Shannon went on to the support
group. "They provided so much help and encouragement for
me, right at the time when the magnitude of what we were up
against had really just hit me. It was a crisis time for me—and
they just surrounded me with caring support."

That's why it's so crucial to be there, both consistently
and at points of crisis, for both the cancer patient and the family. We never know when an opportune moment for providing
desperately needed encouragement might come along. We cannot know what information may have just been given to the person prior to the time we make that telephone call or visit.

Shannon recalled her group as being there for her, being
sensitive, being available, willing to listen. "They listened to
me, both then and at other times, while I just poured out my
feelings. And so did my friends. Annie, my spiritual mom. Kim,
my college roommate. They were there for me, time and again.

"And Jack Taylor was there for Jim. He and Jim had been
in seminary together. Jack would come to Houston periodically
to visit Jim and Jamie Buckingham, who was also hospitalized
in Houston for cancer—at M.D. Anderson. Jack was an incredible encourager from both Jim and Jamie. He even taught us
about different spiritual issues too, like prayer and spiritual
warfare. You know, you never get to the point where you can't
continue to learn. But Jack taught us in such a supportive fash-

ion. And he seemed to sense the times when we were ready to learn."

Exercising that kind of discernment is of utmost importance for those who would be supportive of cancer patients and their families. There are optimal times for learning, for reinforcing spiritual truths. There are other times when the thing to do is just to be there and listen. After all, James 1:19 reminds us, "Let every man be swift to hear, slow to speak, slow to wrath." God has given each of us two ears and only one mouth. Perhaps the rule of thumb for encouragement and counseling should be to listen twice as much as we speak.

Shannon recalled that Jack Taylor's sensitivity in listening and being supportive played as big a role as what he taught them. "Both were important. He listened. He supported us. And he taught us. Other colleagues from Rapha and from the *Stress In Ministry* conferences provided encouragement and insight as well. And I learned a lot spiritually from Annie. She kept on reminding me where God was in all of this—I really needed to hear that. It helped keep me from feeling bitter toward God."

One key component of the support offered by Dr. Rodgers was his sense of humor. He was a large man, husky and more than six feet tall with a full head of thick, dark hair. "We always knew when he was coming. We'd hear the sound of his laughter. Now it wasn't like he was a comedian, coming in telling a lot of jokes when he dealt with us. It was just that he was a cheerful man who laughed a lot. And that laughter was encouraging and infectious.

"Our radiologist, Dr. Walker, also had a great sense of humor. As a Christian, he provided us with a lot of encouragement as well. He was in charge of Jim's radiation treatments following his surgery."

Saying Good-bye

Shannon remembered another important incident, one in which Dr. Walker played a role. "It was when they were about to take Jim for the needle biopsy. You know, they leave you waiting in the hallway on a gurney before you go in. Ron Johnson was there with us. Jim looked up at me and said, 'Shannon, I have some things I need to say to you.'"

It was a poignant moment. Jim referenced the film *Always*: "I'll be like Richard Dreyfuss to you. I'll make sure you're taken care of. But you're young. You have a great life ahead of you."

"I remember telling him to shut up. I wasn't ready to hear that," Shannon recalled, her voice strained with emotion. "At that point, we didn't know for absolute certain it was cancer, even though Dr. Rodgers was pretty sure. This was the needle biopsy that would confirm the diagnosis. I felt like, *Where is this coming from? I don't want to hear this.* After all, we were going to beat this thing—no matter what. So I didn't want to hear even a hint about dying. But as I reflect back, Jim was starting to say good-bye to me at that point. And he trusted Ron as a friend so much that he wanted him to hear what he had to say to me."

Because of the intense suffering that made it so difficult for Jim to think or even be there for much of the time during the months between the diagnosis and his death, Shannon now considers that moment to be her actual good-bye from her husband. "Little did I know at that time what we would go through, or how it would all end up. But that really was our farewell. I see God's hand in that. But I also appreciate the encouragement of Ron being there for both of us then—and how he and others were there for us for what we had to face during the days that followed."

Shannon credits Ron and other close friends for helping her process feelings of anger over the pain Jim suffered, both from the cancer and from the many invasive medical procedures that were a part of his battle against the disease. Her voice choked as she admitted, "I guess I still have some anger to deal with. I just hate that Jim had to go through so much. He nearly died in February before we finally lost him in June. But he suffered through so much before he died."

Shannon was quick to point out how her support network had helped her time and again as she had to deal with waves of anger over the whole process. "They were there to listen, to help me, to support me whenever I would get stuck. And I did from time to time—I think any of us do."

When the needle biopsy results came back, everyone's worst fears were confirmed. "It was a fourth level tumor," Shannon recalled. "You can't get much worse than that."

The surgical procedure for pancreatic cancer was extremely risky. Shannon recalled being told that "a lot of people die from the surgery itself." Jim survived the surgery, but it was a difficult ordeal. "There was so much scar tissue—they almost couldn't get to the tumor itself during the operation."

After the Surgery

Following the surgery, Shannon began what would become a regular ordeal of caring for Jim, encouraging him when he was down and depressed or suffering from the intense pain, plus taking care of a seemingly endless number of chores. "The first few months, Jim had a pretty high level of fear. Even though he knew and understood all the biblical truths, and his faith was firm in the Lord, he was still afraid. After his second hospitalization, he experienced more of a peace. But it was an ordeal both for him and for me. Neither of us were the 'stoic Christians' a lot of people expected us to be. It's a good thing we had friends who could allow us both to express anger without condemning us. They provided the support so we could 'be angry and sin not,' like it says in Ephesians 4:26. They listened, and they helped.

When choosing a place for cancer treatment, it is extremely important for cancer patients and family members to factor in the personal support.

"I was so afraid about going home from the hospital that first time. Sure enough, my worst fears were confirmed. We would have home nursing instead of the round-the-clock care you have in the hospital. Insurance just wouldn't pay for twenty-four-hour nursing care, but Jim needed care available around the clock. So I was it—I was the one to give him the injections for pain. Later, when he developed diabetes, I had to give him his insulin injections."

Among Shannon's unpleasant recollections is the way some friends tried to insist on telling them what to do: "You just simply must go to M.D. Anderson. It's the only place you can get good treatment," or, "Try Laetrile" or one of the other alternative treatments.

"But we decided to keep Jim at the hospital near our home. It was an excellent facility, and we both needed the support from having our friends nearby. Even though M.D. Anderson was a great facility, we didn't feel it was the place for us. And we definitely didn't think trying something like Laetrile was the thing to do."

When choosing a place for cancer treatment, it is extremely important for cancer patients and family members to factor in the personal support. "That's especially true," Shannon suggested, "because of the computerized treatment protocols available to doctors all over the country. As an oncologist, Roger had access to the same protocols they would use at M.D. Anderson, Memorial Sloan-Kettering, or anywhere else in the country. And our local hospital had the proper equipment to make those treatments happen."

Jim underwent seven and a half weeks of radiation, plus simultaneous chemotherapy. "Roger had worked at M.D. Anderson for twelve years. He had also been at Clear Lake—our hospital—for the past fourteen years. I felt he was the person to help us sort through both the solicited and unsolicited advice and come up with the best choice. And he did. I feel good about our decision to keep Jim at Clear Lake for treatment, where he and I both had the greatest access to our support network. Roger helped us evaluate all the options. He said, 'If you need to go to Anderson, I'll support you. But there are also reasons to consider having the treatment here.'"

A big factor, according to Shannon, was that "Jim needed the personal care. He needed to know that the people knew him. Not only those treating him, but that he had supportive friends nearby."

Unfortunately, there were still some who, after Shannon and Jim had made their decision, kept insisting, "You've made a big mistake. You're in the wrong place."

"Those kinds of comments really didn't help us at all."

The Value of Support

One of the threads common to everyone we have talked with is the incredible value of supportive family members and friends. For Tom (chapters 1, 5), it was Judith, his administrative assistant, who stood with him throughout his time of treatment. "She was such a jewel—always there for me. Sometimes she'd bug me about keeping on with the treatments whenever I threatened to drop out. But I always knew I could count on her."

For Liz (chapters 2, 7), primary support came from her husband, Bill. "I don't know what I would have done without him. He was such a trooper. When I was constantly up and down, he was as steady as a rock."

For Jessica (chapter 3) and her parents, Ron and Dianna, the prayer, support, presence, encouragement, and help of Christian friends from their church family played a crucial role. "Each time Jessica had major surgery, the church would set up a twenty-four-hour prayer vigil," Ron noted. "People visited with us in the hospital. In fact, at times there were so many people who came just to be with us that the hospital actually had to give us a separate room. And somebody would bring in food— sandwiches for the whole group. They were so supportive."

For Angela (chapter 4), it was her special friend Ginger, the oncology nurse who was "an angel of mercy sent my way. I remember that she was the only person who talked to me and listened to what I had to say. She treated me like a person, not just a cancer patient. She helped me understand what was happening to me. And I never had to be brave for her. She was there whenever I needed her—she went so far beyond the call of duty. I remember her being there to hold my hand when I had a spinal tap."

For Candy (chapter 6), the key support came from her family. "My parents and my husband were so wonderful and supportive. They were there to fluff my pillows and rub my legs. But they couldn't give me real peace or strength. That could only come from the Lord. But it sure made a difference to know they were there for me. Then there was the friend who had done his residency program at the Mayo Clinic, Dr. Raleigh Kemp. He's the one who put me in touch with Dr. Jackson and helped me make arrangements to come to the Mayo Clinic for the surgery that ultimately saved my life."

According to Cliff (chapters 3, 8), the majority of his human support came from his wife, Gloria, and from his oldest son, Arnie. "All my family provided me with so much help and strength. Gloria was there to drive me to therapy, and even to listen to me when I griped. And Arnie seemed to have wisdom and insight far beyond his years—he's in pre-med now and plans to be a doctor. I think he'll make a great one. I know my ultimate trust is in God, but He sure used my family to bring me through this time."

Practical Steps

So how can you go about supporting a friend or relative who has been diagnosed with cancer? How do you encourage and support the family members? The basic thrust is to provide encouragement. Encouragement is the biblical process "prompted by love" and "directed toward fear."[2] The common emotional thread running beneath the variety of emotions experienced by the cancer patient and the patient's family is fear. The biblical encourager applies God's unconditional love to help relieve that fear.

Don't be afraid to bring up the subject of cancer.

Some of the following principles have already been stated but need to be considered again for emphasis. Although the steps listed are not exhaustive, they are the ones we consider most important for extending encouragement.

1 *Make contact.* As Shannon Mahoney so clearly explained, "Don't tell someone, 'Call me if you need me.' They never will. Just come. Get involved. Find ways to help. I remember so many times when Ron Johnson would come by to pick Jim up to take him to his radiation therapy. That freed me to take care of the things that needed to be done around the house, and have a few moments just for myself, without the pressure of taking care of Jim. Then someone from Rapha provided a pager, and someone else a portable phone. Then there were a number of people who came and helped with the overwhelming amount of laundry. Our friends sort of organized to help with those kinds of things. They also helped by picking up prescriptions and other supplies at the drugstore."

2 *Establish appropriate communication* that includes supportive, life-giving words to share honest comfort and positive
cheer. An important component of such communication is listening, but it also involves speaking the truth in love (Ephesians
4:15) as well as being "swift to hear, slow to speak" (James
1:19). Sometimes the best thing to do is to take the person away
from the situation for a cup of coffee, a time away, a chance to
talk. At other times, staying at the scene with them is best.

And don't be afraid to bring up the subject of cancer. As
Shannon observed, "A time or two, people would come to visit
Jim and me and never ask how he was doing. Never even mention his cancer. I'm sure it was awkward. But I know how it
helped me to have people bring up the subject and to ask how
we were doing."

There does come a time when good friends need to inter-
vene, to simply step in, either individually or as a group at a
point of crisis. Shannon faced such a point shortly after she and
Jim returned from their first stay in the hospital.

"We were home, and I was trying to carry the whole load.
I felt so overwhelmed. I was not getting any rest. Then there was
a horrible Saturday night, when Jim was in incredible pain and
intensely depressed. The next day, Sunday, our friend Delvin
drove over. He and his wife, Carolyn, were such good friends,
they stayed with us the whole day. Dixon and Lois, our friends
from *Stress In Ministry* conferences, and Roger and Annie came
over as well. I didn't know what I was going to do. But it was
like the whole group just intervened. They told me, 'Shannon,
you can't handle this.' Jim was in such bad shape, and I was the
only one helping. I don't think I would have survived much
longer if things had gone on like they were."

With Jim's physical and emotional condition having left
Shannon, his primary support, at the point of despair, the group
insisted that Dr. Roger Rodgers be contacted and arrangements
made to return Jim to the hospital. "I don't think it would be a
stretch to say that their intervention saved me. I knew things
were at the point where I couldn't go on. But I didn't want to
admit it. My friends helped me admit it—and also helped me
find a way out."

3 *Help the cancer patient and the family evaluate and take
advantage of resources.* A cancer support group can be one
of the most important resources. "I remember the first one I

attended—the stories I heard just about wiped me out," Shannon related. "But the printed resources, the caring people, the contact person whose name I was given—that support group experience really opened my eyes. Cancer support groups aren't for everyone. But for many patients and families, they provide an invaluable resource."

At its most basic level, a support group is any two or more people who are willing and able to provide emotional or physical help. However, a support group generally refers to an organized group that meets regularly to deal with a common issue. The local office of the American Cancer Society or most hospitals that treat cancer can provide information on cancer support groups.

Support groups can provide a great deal of insight and information, a network of encouragement and help, and a safe place to talk about the fears and emotions related to cancer. However, some people find attending a support group to be difficult—or even devastating. At times those who attend will find themselves discouraged or overwhelmed, when they see and hear from people who are worse off than they are or hear reactions to a person's specific situation, like those experienced by Shannon when she explained that her husband had pancreatic cancer. She recalled painfully how some people had responded with remarks about how pancreatic cancer left a patient with almost no hope. "They were telling the truth—but it was just devastating to me."

Shannon believes that two types of cancer support groups are needed: "One for the immediacy of finding out about cancer treatment resources. Then perhaps another one for the long haul." Shannon also suggested encouraging families to take advantage of technology, such as the beeper Rapha provided so that she could stay in touch with Jim when she was out of the house. "Someone also furnished a portable telephone, which Jim kept right beside him. Eventually, when he became sicker, we purchased a baby monitor—that was very helpful because it allowed me to get some sleep in my own bed but still be available. They have two settings, one where you can hear everything, and another where you can hear only louder things, like a call for help. With that setting, I felt comfortable going to sleep, knowing that Jim had a way to wake me if he needed me. That's the kind of thing a person could just purchase and give or loan the cancer patient or the family."

Another tangible means of encouragement is to provide financial assistance. Barnabas, one of the great encouragers of the New Testament, demonstrated his willingness to encourage by providing for those in the church who were facing intense financial struggles. He actually sold his family property to help meet the needs of Christian friends (Acts 4:36–37). Shannon reported that there were many who contributed in this way to assist her and Jim. Ron Eggert's experience during Jessica's treatment paralleled that of the Mahoneys. "We had so many incidental expenses beyond insurance and medical coverage. Meals at the hospital, travel back and forth. There were so many people who gave, some a little, some a lot—but it all helped immeasurably."

Shannon recalled how the financial help of others was so crucial because "often you have to wait for reimbursement from insurance companies on medications, and everything is so expensive." Some even provided bundles of washcloths and towels, and someone provided Jim with a lightweight wheelchair. "It let us get out of the house, go shopping, do a lot of things together that Jim couldn't do because he had been so weakened by the cancer. I couldn't handle the weight of a standard-size chair. But the lightweight wheelchair was just what we needed."

4 Another important element of emotional support is to *allow people the freedom to cry.* Such freedom usually exists in support groups. It is crucial that Christian friends and family members allow this as well. "There were many times when tears just came," Shannon said. "They were essential to allow Jim and me to handle the intense emotions we were feeling. Our circle of friends provided a climate of acceptance in which it was OK for us to cry—and they wept with us. They were true examples of what it means to weep with those who weep."

Unfortunately, there are still some Christians today who advocate the stiff-upper-lip mentality—that it is a sign of Christian weakness to weep. Somehow they overlook Paul's injunction to "rejoice with those who rejoice, and weep with those who weep" (Romans 12:15). They miss the stark yet compassionate picture painted by the terse wording of John in his observation that "Jesus wept" (John 11:35). And they ignore David's perspective on God's compassionate evaluation of our tears: "You number my wanderings; put my tears into Your bottle; are they not in Your book?" (Psalm 56:8). Certainly the picture painted by the psalmist of God collecting teardrops in the leather bottles of that day stands as a graphic reminder that, since God allows and encourages appropriate tears, God's people should as well.

5 Finally, *seek to communicate realistic hope.* Shannon recalls the response of many people who, although they didn't come out and use words such as *terminal,* would indicate by their expressions how hopeless they considered Jim's situation to be. Sometimes an encouraging word, a card, a note, or even a book sharing positive encouragement, perhaps from someone who has survived cancer, can help counter the feelings of hopelessness that so commonly affect the cancer patient and the family.

It is essential to convey to young family members a positive, yet balanced, hope. Shannon suggests, "Be honest. Tell children. Not every detail. And be careful about how you explain God's part. Using phrases like 'God's going to take Daddy home' can really leave a child with a long-term struggle with bitterness toward God." As a therapist and the spouse of someone who battled cancer, Shannon suggests, "It's best to let the child bring up any question about death. But be ready. It probably will come up. And be careful when death does occur not to couch your attempted encouragement in words that leave children or adults blaming God. After all, hope has to be balanced. It's important to encourage people to hope for the best, yet be prepared for the worse."

Experts say that if you do not tell children of cancer patients anything, their imagination may actually lead them to conclusions that produce fears much worse than the actual situation. Also, remember that children pick up as much by *how* you say it as by *what* you actually say.

Sickness, suffering, and death are integral parts of the human experience. But for the Christian, the reality of the resurrection of Christ provides a solid basis for hope beyond death. The Christian encourager can seek to instill hope without conveying expectations that the cancer patient or the family must handle things a certain way.

Shannon gives the highest marks to those who consistently encouraged her. "I'm just so grateful for those individuals who helped bolster my spirits. They didn't expect me to perform. They were there with me in every crisis and in the routine. They were willing to wash dishes, clean bathrooms, run to the drug store, whatever needed to be done."

Accepting Help

Supportive friends offering help is only part of the equation. The other element involves cancer patients and families accepting help. For some individuals, accepting help is extremely difficult. Perhaps they have been taught or conditioned from childhood never to ask for help, to be self-reliant.

Yet cancer piles intense emotional pressure on top of the physical stress caused by the disease. Plus the typical cancer treatment regimen demands a great deal of time and energy itself. That's why it's important for the cancer patient and the family to be willing to accept help. Allowing others to run errands, help with cleaning, cook meals, and do other routine chores can let the patient and the family devote more time and energy to dealing with the cancer, making important decisions, and getting the best medical care. Cooking meals, providing transportation—including getting children to school, music lessons, sporting events, or doctor or dentist appointments— housekeeping chores, shopping, baby-sitting, or helping deal with the minor crises of life such as automotive breakdown are just a few of the forms such help can take.

For many people, accepting help is uncomfortable enough. Asking for help is even worse. Recognizing the biblical principle that "it is more blessed to give than to receive" (Acts 20:35), it is appropriate to allow others the blessing of giving to us. Developing a list of needs, then communicating those needs to people who call or visit and offer to help, can be one way to overcome the unease some people feel. Family members, close friends, or even casual acquaintances from church or work may be eager to provide help. When these sources are unable to provide sufficient assistance, sometimes the medical treatment team, or even a social worker, can provide information about available resources and help. It is important to give people the opportunity to help by communicating needs. Remember, people cannot read our minds.

The network of loving friends and family members can also help the cancer patient and the family cope with the added stress cancer brings to the relationship. As Shannon explained, "Jim's cancer produced a strain on our marriage like we had never experienced. The two of us just didn't have enough support to give, to be able to just lean on each other. We needed our supportive friends through those tough times, both individually and for our relationship."

Even the best of marriages, friendships, or family relationships will be strained by the added stress produced by cancer and its effects. Fatigue is a key factor. A variety of fears tend to multiply like weeds in a springtime garden. Roles change, leading to confusion and frustration. An extra measure of the fruit of the Spirit—love, joy, peace, longsuffering, kindness, goodness, faithfulness, gentleness, and self-control—can go a long way for the victim and the family, as well as for those extending support and help.

10

LIVING WITH CANCER, DYING OF CANCER

D o you sometimes get the impression that cancer is permeating our society, forcing its way into every arena of life?
There are times when it seems that way. Newspaper stories
carry accounts of famous people who succumb to cancer: Au-
drey Hepburn, actress and humanitarian, dead at sixty-three of
colon cancer; Chuck Connors, two-sport professional athlete,
known best for his role as television's "Rifleman," dead at seventy-one of lung cancer.

Magazines carry the story of the impact of this dreaded
complex of diseases. Even as the 1992 presidential campaign of
incumbent George Bush floundered toward defeat, senior Republican political strategists played the "What if?" game,
mourning the loss the year before of Republican National Committee Chairman Lee Atwater, who died of brain cancer at forty.
A feature article in *People* magazine focused on Lee's widow,
Sally, who told reporters, "There's not a minute that goes by
that I don't think about him."[1]

The first two out of three 1993 issues of *Sports Illustrated*
seemed to focus as much on cancer as on athletic competition.
In the January 11 issue, a feature story on college-basketball-
coach-turned-broadcaster Jim Valvano's fight with cancer
eclipsed the story of Alabama's victory over Miami for college
football's national championship. Two weeks later, the January

25 issue carried the story of hockey great Mario Lemieux, diagnosed with Hodgkin's disease the previous week by doctors in Pittsburgh. Despite Lemieux's and his doctor's prediction of a complete recovery, *SI* writer Jon Scher noted that "his life, not to mention his extraordinary career, hangs in the balance."[2] Ironically, the article about Lemieux reminded readers that, little more than a year before, Bob Johnson, who had coached the Pittsburgh Penguins to the first of two consecutive Stanley Cup championships, died of brain cancer. The year before that, Pittsburgh goalie Tom Barrasso's two-year-old daughter, Ashley, barely survived a bout with neuroblastoma, a deadly form of childhood cancer. For a time it almost seemed that the editors of *Sports Illustrated* were trading articles with the *New England Journal of Medicine*.

Living with cancer. Dying of cancer. It's becoming far more common than any of us would like to think. We hear about it from a colleague at the office, a friend at church, aunts, uncles, cousins, children, and parents. We see the pictures in the papers—the glamorous-looking photo of twenty-one-year-old Jennifer, whose obituary reads, "[She] left us after a courageous eighteen-month battle with cancer October second." Or the story of young Guerrero who, according to his relatives, "lived up to his name, which means beloved warrior, in his fight with leukemia." Guerrero died at the age of fourteen at Baylor University Medical Center. These pictures and obituaries, printed one October morning in the *Dallas Morning News*, and thousands of others like them, don't begin to capture the horror, the devastation, the incredible impact cancer produces.

> *One out of three people*
> *who have been diagnosed with cancer*
> *have been pronounced cured.*

Cancer knows no social, political, economic, or spiritual barriers. Rachel Tyrell died of lung cancer at fifty-one after a career that included a college professorship in English literature, membership in the international English Honors Society, civic activity in the junior league, and membership in the Dallas Shakespeare Festival Board of Directors. *USA Today* printed the obituary of eighty-two-year-old Dorothy Hawkins, who died in

Birmingham, Alabama, after decades of work with the Alabama Eye Foundation, the local eye bank, the local tumor registry, and various other medical, civic, and charitable causes.

Cancer has cut short the lives of many of God's choicest servants in the spiritual arena. Countless thousands of Christians were touched by the writing and speaking ministry of Christian apologist Francis Schaeffer, who died May 15, 1984, after an extended bout with cancer. Dr. James Mahoney (story in chapter 9), who helped Robert McGee found Rapha Treatment Centers in 1986, died of cancer early in 1991.

Approximately one million new cases of cancer are diagnosed each year in the United States.[3] On the other side of the coin, nearly two million Americans are considered cured of cancer today, still alive more than five years after their initial diagnosis and treatment. Overall, one out of three people who have been diagnosed with cancer have been pronounced cured.[4]

Many people live with cancer. Some of them will ultimately die of it. Still others will recover. And God alone knows who fits into which category. As Director of Clinical Research at Baylor University Medical Center, Dr. Stephen Jones has signed many death certificates. One of those was for Debbie Burke, lawyer, wife, mother, and believer. Debbie died when she was thirty-nine, following a second recurrence of breast cancer, which had first appeared five years earlier. Debbie's husband, Casey—tall, with dark hair and an engaging smile—met Debbie while on a business trip from his home in Dallas to Tulsa. He remembered Dr. Jones as normally stoic. "But the day before she died, Dr. Jones looked across the bed at me—I think he was really shaken that day. He said, 'Casey, I did everything I could.'"

At her funeral, Casey, reading from a letter he had written for the occasion, put into perspective how Debbie had lived with, then died of, cancer.

> It's easy for a husband to talk about how sweet and special his wife was, or is—especially in this situation. And Debbie was uniquely special, as you all know. . . . But what I want you all to know is that the grace and courage that she displayed during the last few years of her battle were epitomized these last few weeks of her life. And even though her body literally destroyed itself, her

spirit became more and more beautiful. And the power of God has never been more apparent to me.

Debbie died for a lot of reasons—for each person who was so deeply touched and changed by her, for the people who came to Christ, and who will come to Christ because of her—and to make me a man of God.

Tall and statuesque, with a full head of flowing straw-berry-blonde hair, sparkling green eyes, a dusting of freckles across her light complexion, a cheerful sense of humor and a quick wit, Debbie had set out to fulfill her lifelong goal of becoming a lawyer. Ironically, receiving her law degree from the University of Tulsa School of Law and passing her bar exam were two of her final achievements before she lost her final battle with cancer. Her husband remembered Debbie as "a caring person and extremely organized. She was the kind of person I could easily fall in love with and marry—and I did." After a courtship that lasted a little more than a year, the two finally tied the marital knot in the fall of 1987.

By the time Casey and Debbie married, the cancer had already made its presence felt in Debbie's body. On July 2, 1986, her right breast had to be removed following the discovery of a malignant lump. Casey related how both their lives were forever changed.

"In June 1986, I was scheduled to go on a business trip to Switzerland. The day before I left she called. She had been to the doctor after finding a lump some weeks before. She hadn't told me about it—she didn't want to worry me. I was at the office when she called. She told me she had already had a biopsy. That they had discovered a lump in her breast. And that she had cancer. I remember sitting there at my desk, and just caving in.

"My immediate response, even though I was to leave the next morning for a twelve-hour flight to Switzerland, was to grab the next plane from Dallas to Tulsa. At that point, we weren't actually engaged, but we loved each other. We grieved, we cried together—and she insisted that I go ahead with the trip to Switzerland. She had a great medical team, plus the support of her family, and the doctors told us she was in a very high survivability category.

"I remember the surgeon, Dr. John Frame, discussing the options of mastectomy versus lumpectomy with Debbie and me. When I asked him, he said without hesitation, 'If this were my wife, facing the same circumstances, the mastectomy is the procedure I'd choose.' I had absolutely no problem with that. Debbie's choice to have the mastectomy never bothered me as a husband—I never thought any less of her because of the surgery. From my perspective, her femininity wasn't diminished in the least."

Radical Change

From the point of Debbie's diagnosis of cancer, just as with countless other cancer victims, life would never be the same again. A part of her body had to be surgically removed, leaving her with a very obvious change. She and her husband would be reminded of the change literally every day for the rest of their lives. Other forms of cancer may not bring about quite as drastic or as obvious a change. Nonetheless, the changes are there.

For forty-six-year-old Jim Valvano life had been filled with winning a national men's collegiate basketball championship at North Carolina State University, then becoming a respected television analyst at ABC and ESPN. But when he was diagnosed with metastatic adenocarcinoma, his life was altered drastically. As he put it, "I travel a different world now. I'm in the world of terminal illness."[5] He says cancer changed his life more than any other factor, including the height of winning a national championship and the depth of losing his job in the wake of an athletic department scandal.

It had started with what seemed a little thing—an ache in his crotch. Then came the response of the radiologist at Duke University following an MRI and comparison of the views taken of his spine with those of a healthy person. Jim had cancer. Suddenly, completely, irreversibly, life had been changed.

Though cancer is listed second to cardiovascular disease as the leading cause of death among adults in our society—taking 184 per 100,000 population—everyone dies sooner or later. And to die, you have to be alive in the first place. So, in a sense, you could say that the leading cause of death is life.[6] Although death is a common appointment for every human being, it is the uncertainly regarding the time of the cancer patient's death, coupled with the knowledge of the kind of death cancer frequently causes and the profound changes to daily life it brings, that so greatly upsets the life of the cancer patient.

The foundation of a vital faith can help the cancer patient, as well as those closest to him or her, cope with the incredible upheaval brought on by a cancer diagnosis. Debbie Burke had such faith. "She had come to faith as a child," Casey remembered. He had trusted Christ at thirteen. After Debbie's cancer diagnosis and surgery in July 1986 and their marriage in September of the following year, "We sensed that the only option we had was to lean on God to walk us through whatever lay ahead. We were able to encourage each other and to grow spiritually as a result."

The thought of cancer was never far from the minds of Debbie and Casey. That's how it is when individuals have cancer. It becomes a form of bondage.

The year following their marriage, Spencer was born—the doctors anticipated no problem with the pregnancy from Debbie's cancer. "Even the decision about having a baby necessitated our consulting with Debbie's cancer doctor," Casey recalled. "Even when we thought things were going well, that she had the cancer licked, we still had to take it into account. When you have the kind of surgery Debbie had, you go back every three months for a couple of years. Then if everything's OK, they move you to every six months. We didn't really think much about the cancer recurring—we certainly weren't cancer paranoid. Perhaps it was the nature of both our personalities. We had faith in the Lord, we had done everything we knew to do, and we had positive assurances from Dr. Frame."

Yet the thought of cancer was never far from the minds of Debbie and Casey. That's how it is when individuals have cancer. It becomes a form of bondage. That's what happened to Nancy, who was diagnosed with acute leukemia. When the forty-five-year-old saw her doctor because of fatigue and shortness of breath, she had a successful marriage, a career of her own, and two children. Nancy didn't think she had time for cancer. In fact, her initial reaction was denial.

Within a few days, she was hospitalized. Questions concerning diagnosis were followed by confirmation. After her initial hospitalization, Nancy returned to the doctor every two weeks to have her white cell count monitored in order to track her response. During her extended chemotherapy, Nancy's hair began falling out in large clumps. Because of her susceptibility to infection, she had to watch carefully for skin lesions and take extra care of her mouth.

It was three weeks after her second hospitalization before Nancy was able to return home. According to a bone marrow test, intensive chemotherapy appeared to have wiped out the leukemic cells. Her oncologist established a maintenance program of chemotherapy, and she learned to give herself injections of a variety of drugs. Several of the medications produced nausea and vomiting, making it almost impossible for Nancy to carry on even routine activities such as visiting friends or buying groceries at the local supermarket. Radically, irreversibly, Nancy's life had been changed by cancer.

Life on Hold

As Casey described the changes that came about in his life with Debbie, he talked about trying to counter what he called the disruption factor. "I work for a Swiss watch manufacturer, spending a lot of time on the road calling on clients. Cancer just destroys your routine. I'm a road man, and there were many weeks I just couldn't go on the road.

"We found so much of our life taken up by cancer—going for treatments, spending time in the hospital, learning things about cancer and how to treat it, things I never planned on learning." Casey recalled a time during the course of Debbie's treatment when, following a discussion of a variety of medications with the treatment team in Dr. Jones's office, he walked out into the hallway with Dr. Jim Hagins. "When I began quoting back to him the drugs we had discussed—adriamyacin, methotrexate, and several others, Jim seemed surprised. He said, 'Casey, you sure have learned a lot.' To which I replied, 'Yeah, about a lot of things I wish I knew nothing about.'

"But the longer we went with Debbie's cancer, the more I learned—and the greater the effect of the cancer on Debbie. I guess there's a sense in which, being in the business I am, working with watches, I could see Debbie's body sort of winding down like a watch.

"There were three times when you could say news about Debbie's cancer sort of kicked us in the stomach. There was that first time, before we were married, when she called me from Tulsa the day before I flew to Switzerland.

"The second time was after our marriage. I was on the road—in Tulsa, ironically. Debbie was back in Dallas, where, at SMU, she was able to finish some of the work on her law degree." Casey recalled being in a client's store when he received a surprise phone call from Debbie—"She always knew where to find me." She told him she was OK, warned him not to worry, "but I have cancer again."

"It was just as shocking as it was the first time—the bottom just fell out all over again. I remember it was raining—miserable weather. I had a four-and-a-half-hour drive home to Dallas. Outside the rain was pouring down. In the car, I cried all the way. It was like I felt my gut squeezed inside out. "It was the longest few hours I'd ever spent—although there were a lot longer hours to come."

When Casey arrived back in Dallas, Debbie was at home, surrounded by friends from their Bible study class. A few minutes after he arrived, the doorbell rang. "It was Pastor Steve. He came in, knelt between Debbie and me, and prayed. I remember tangibly sensing God's presence and taking hope at that point. It was a very special time."

For Debbie and Casey there were two major concerns: *Could* she finish law school, and *should* she? And what about Spencer? "Debbie's major concern was our one-year-old son. At this point we were beginning to at least consider the possibility that she wouldn't make it. The one thing that really seemed to trouble her was leaving our child with no mommy. That really bothered her, probably more than anything."

Then there was the matter of law school. When the doctors said her cancer had returned, Debbie needed two semesters to earn her law degree. Despite undergoing intense chemotherapy, she managed to complete those final two semesters to earn her degree, then pass the bar exam. Casey remembered discussing with Debbie whether she should worry about completing law school while fighting the cancer. "We just never considered this as some kind of waste of money, or that she might not live to use it. Debbie was so goal-oriented, to do anything different than finish up would not have been her. She really didn't change a lot in terms of her personality—who she was."

Loss of Hair

Among the life-change factors mentioned by almost every cancer patient is the loss of hair, a frequent result of either chemotherapy or radiation therapy. "That was a big one for Debbie," Casey recalled. "You try to convince yourself, 'Oh, it's not important.' But it really is. Her strawberry-blonde hair was so beautiful, so unusual, and such a distinctive part of her physical appearance. At first, she had all her hair—it looked normal. Then it began to gradually fall out. Finally it became so thin she really worked at the creative use of scarves and hats.

"Then it was all gone. At that point she began to wear the wigs she had purchased for this very thing. I remember thinking, *What a shame. Her natural hair was so beautiful, and now she's forced into wearing fake hair.*" But Debbie persevered with her treatment. Months of chemo brought her back to the point where the doctors said, "It looks like you're cancer free."

Casey recalled a special party with thirty or more friends at Culpepper's—a steak-and-ribs restaurant located near the shore of Lake Ray Hubbard, just east of Dallas. "We called it her 'Celebration of Life.' She had finished law school and her chemo. We were ready to get on with life. It was a great occasion, a special opportunity to say thank you to our close friends, and to affirm to ourselves, each other, and those who stood with us that we had this thing licked. So we celebrated and tried to put the cancer thing behind us. But we'd already been through the emotional crash twice. From this point on, those three-month checkups became pretty nerve-racking."

Facing our mortality isn't easy. For the cancer patient and his or her family, it's essential. Martin Luther once told his followers, "Even in the best of health we should have death always before our eyes, so that we will not expect to remain on this earth forever, but will have one foot in the air so to speak."[7]

There's a sense in which, for those who have cancer, life boils down to two major issues: first, survival; second, preparation for death. Sometimes these two objectives are so intertwined as to be difficult to separate. Prior to his own untimely death, not from cancer but at the hands of hostile natives, Jim Elliot told his wife Elizabeth, "Wherever you are, be all there. Live to the hilt each day what you believe to be the will of God."[8]

One of the decisions Casey and Debbie made was to not quit living, despite the threat of cancer. Not only would she complete her law degree, she would sit for the bar exam. And she "passed with flying colors." Then the two of them planned "the trip of a lifetime" to celebrate—two weeks in Europe. Casey gave it to Debbie as "sort of a present for finishing law school." It turned out to be the last trip of Debbie's life.

Casey recalled their flying into Frankfurt, Germany, renting a car, spending several days with friends Debbie had met fifteen years before. "She had met these people in Shreveport. They were from Heidelberg. And she had kept up with them, written to them. She was that kind of person. You know, some of us meet people and promise to write, then never do. But Debbie had written them. She kept in touch."

---

*Up to 40 percent of cancer patients
do not receive enough medication
to control their pain.*

After spending two days with those friends, Debbie and Casey drove through the Black Forest region of southern Germany, then into Switzerland and Austria. Yet even as they enjoyed the incredible scenery and adventure of the trip, Debbie began to experience persistent pain in her shoulder. Both of them feared the worst.

"We kept praying. Kept talking about it. Hoping nothing was wrong. But in the back of my mind—I knew. She did, too."

From that point on, two major factors seemed to dominate Debbie's life, and Casey's—pain and prayer. "During the trip, and on the way back, we prayed our guts out. But she just kept hurting worse and worse. More and more. The pain was the dominating factor on the trip, especially toward the end."

The Pain Factor

Pain became a major factor in Jim Valvano's life as well. His back hurt, his hips, his knees. Sometimes as many as twenty-four tablets of Advil were necessary to get him through each painful day.

A Reuters news release suggested that up to 40 percent of cancer patients do not receive enough medication to control their pain.[9] A study of 1,200 patients in outpatient clinics suggested that the problem is especially acute for women under fifty—this according to Dr. Charles Cleeland, Director of the Pain Research Group at the University of Wisconsin Medical School. Women under fifty and older patients tend to receive less potent medication, even when the patients say they are experiencing significant pain.

According to Dr. Cleeland, poor communication is one reason doctors may underprescribe potent pain killers. Physicians do not routinely ask patients specific questions about pain. In turn, many patients are reluctant to complain. "Debbie didn't have that problem, though," Casey noted. "She was mentally tough. She could handle the thing about dying—had a grip on facing death—except for leaving our son behind. But the physical pain was another story. At times it would really get to her."

For Jim Valvano, projecting physical toughness was important. He often refused to take his prescription pain pills. But the constant need was there for more and more Advil, as the pain kept increasing.

Yet pain isn't exclusive to cancer patients. All of us hurt to some degree. Evidence indicates that babies experience pain even before birth. Then life is filled with one pain after another from the moment of birth till the last struggle for that final breath. There is pain on the outside—pain from a cut, from a broken wrist, from arthritis, from bumping your head on a car door. There is also the reality of inner pain—the pain that comes from life's hurts, abuses, disappointments, and grief.

Like physical pain, emotional pain can draw us inexorably toward addiction to whatever offers relief. As Robert McGee, founder and President of Rapha Treatment Centers, suggests in his booklet *Dealing with Pain,* "Man's way to handle [pain] . . . is to become addicted to some process which can bring release. In fact, the faster release is found, the more seductive is the process used. And the faster the process man uses to reduce pain, the more addictive it becomes."[10] That's why we say heroin is more addictive than many other chemical substances. It works faster.

No one likes pain. Counselors like Robert McGee hate to see individuals struggling to cope with the incredible emotional pain caused by childhood trauma or sexual abuse or the agonizing certainty that death is imminent, leaving only the question of how much suffering will take place first.

For Debbie Burke, after returning from Europe, her body wracked with pain, sitting in a doctor's office, clasping Casey's hand, pain had become an intense, pervasive reality. Likewise for Jim Valvano, canceling an appearance on an ESPN sports program and a weekend of activities because the pain was so overwhelming. From this comes a logical question: What should be our response to pain?

There are two extremes to which we can go. Neither is appropriate. On the one hand, some people try to practice pain denial. "No, it doesn't hurt," they say through gritted teeth, their words giving evidence to the stoic lie. "Christian's don't hurt" or "Big boys don't cry" they believe. Yet pain is real. It cannot be denied. Its purpose is to somehow signal us, to let us know that something is seriously wrong. Like the warning siren of an automotive security system, pain demands our attention.

Pain is a signal, not to draw attention to itself but to help us see the real, underlying problem. Unfortunately, the other extreme is to immediately look for a way to kill all the pain, get rid of it completely, make it never come back. Robert McGee cautions against

> making God the great pain killer. Those who demand this of God feel betrayed when He doesn't take away their pain with a snap of His fingers. They then feel betrayed by Him—and, like tossing out a bottle of medicine that doesn't work, they throw Him away. You see, God does not say, "Taste of me and see how I zap you out of your problems."[11]

The verse Robert McGee parodied says, "Taste and see that the Lord is good" (Psalm 34:8). When life hurts, the goodness of God becomes the central, focal issue. When pain is present, physical or emotional, I am not to ignore it or deny it. Nor must I allow it to become my focus. Rather, the pain must become a catalyst to force me to look at my situation, my circumstances, from God's perspective.

As many as eighty million people in the United States suffer from chronic pain.

We need to recognize two important principles Casey Burke referred to as "God's right hand and His left hand": "In His right hand is the power to do anything—He certainly has the ability to heal anyone. And He could have removed Debbie's cancer instantly. I certainly asked Him to do so, plenty of times. But His left hand held the plan—and I didn't know the details of the plan. Couldn't, in fact. So I had to trust both His power and His plan."

The apostle Paul recognized that painful circumstances had brought him literally to the point of death (2 Corinthians 1:8–9; 4:8–11). For the apostle to bear up under the crushing reality of impending death, two essentials were necessary.

First, he discovered resources for living one day at a time in dependence on God: "Even though our outward man is perishing, yet the inward man is being renewed day by day" (4:16). For Paul, as for Debbie and Casey, pain had become a chronic, constant part of life. According to some estimates, as many as eighty million people in the United States suffer from chronic pain,[12] many from cancer.

"Debbie was in a lot of pain," Casey recalled. "During those last months, it kept her from sleeping at night. We brought in a hospital bed to try to help her get comfortable. But nothing, not a hospital bed, not the strongest pain medicines, could completely get rid of her pain." That's why for Debbie and Casey, when her physical pain and the emotional pain both of them shared seemed overwhelming, they just had to shift their focus.

That's precisely what Paul found it necessary to do as he sought to cope with the gnawing pain of his day-to-day life. Paul explained his shift in focus this way:

> For our light affliction, which is but for a moment, is working for us a far more exceeding and eternal way of glory, while we do not look at the things which are seen, but at the things which are not seen. For the things which are seen are temporary, but the things which are not seen are eternal. For this we know that if our earthly house, this tent, is destroyed, we have a building from God, a house not made with hands, eternal in the heavens. (4:17–5:1)

Even taking life a day at a time, claiming God's grace to renew his strength in the face of pain and adversity, Paul must have felt overwhelmed. The key to coping with his circumstances was to shift his focus, to consider his overwhelming personal circumstances as light, momentary affliction compared to the benefits eternity held. The word translated "look" (*skopos*) in 2 Corinthians 4:18 is not the usual word. It is an extremely focused term from which we derive the English word *scope.* Anyone who has used a microscope, a telescope, or even the scope on a rifle, can understand what Paul is getting at. A scope allows an individual to focus either on what is very small or is located at a great distance. It allows for an extremely selective focus.

That is precisely what Paul was doing in his circumstances, selectively focusing on eternal reality. He was still aware of the pain of his day-to-day life and the danger of death. But he chose not to focus on "the things which are seen." Rather, his focus was on eternal "things which are not seen." The use of the metaphor "thorn in the flesh" (2 Corinthians 12:7) suggests that Paul lived with daily, chronic pain. To cope with this pain, Paul focused his awareness on the certain knowledge that God had prepared for him a body and a life free from pain—and without end (5:1). Such knowledge remained central in his focus and stirred his emotions (5:2–4). And God's spirit within gave him confidence and strength to "walk by faith, not by sight" (v. 7), focused on the eternal.

Casey remembered vividly the day when he and Debbie began to experience that focus on eternity. It happened on a dark, rainy, gray November afternoon when they walked into the physician's office at Baylor to hear the news that Debbie's cancer had recurred—again. The doctor came right to the point: "Debbie, there's something on your breast bone. We have to do a bone scan."

Casey and Debbie left the office in shock. "We got in our car, just sat there parked on the street outside the office. It was drizzling, and we sat there for the longest time, holding each other, crying together." It was at that point that God broke through Casey's thinking with a reminder of the ultimate hope, the only answer in the face of suffering and death.

"I cried and cried when I looked at Debbie. And then it was like the words just popped into my mouth. I said, 'I wish Jesus would come back right now.' I knew that was the only relief for the way both of us felt."

That special moment of remembering the reality of the believer's blessed hope, that focus beyond the pain to the eternal, became a constant reminder over the next eight months before Debbie was to enter the presence of the Lord. Both of them would return to the memory of that moment "like it was a landmark or a lighthouse. We were already both beginning to grieve. At times the pain for Debbie, and even for me, would seem overwhelming. When those times came, one of us would remind the other of what I had said, sitting in the car. And we both really felt it—we really wished Jesus would come back." It's not surprising that the Christian's hope would provide an anchor for the soul in such a time of suffering and grief.

Dying in Grief

In recent years, a great deal has been written on the subject of grief, the normal response to the experience and perception of loss of a significant person or object.[13] Any loss can produce a grief response—the death of a close friend, the loss of a job, an accident or breakdown that takes away your car. Even the loss of an opportunity can bring about a grief response. Put simply, loss produces grief. As Billy Graham explained, "Grief is universal. It is the method of handling grief that is unique and personal."[14]

For Casey and Debbie, as for most who face what we have come to euphemistically refer to as "terminal cancer," the grieving process actually begins even before the prospect of death has come into conscious thought or discussion. "We had both been thinking about it for a long time," Casey recalled. "We just didn't use the D word. I remember one night about a month before she died—Debbie had such a horrible time. I was beside myself because I couldn't help her. There was no relief from the pain. She couldn't rest. Finally, we were able to get in touch with the doctor. We brought her into the hospital. When he came in to see her later that day, he took me into the hallway and said, 'You just have to face it, Casey. Your wife is dying.' It was the first time Dr. Jones had used the D word."

But Casey had known—known as Debbie struggled with the pain, as he tried to help her get comfortable at night, as he cleaned and dressed the gaping, two-inch, open sore on Debbie's chest, a constant reminder of the malignant cells that were eating away at her vitality. "We didn't give up hope—even up until the very end. We kept praying for miracles. And there were plenty of people who told us miracles would come. We had to keep hoping for the best, trusting God, asking Him for a miracle. But we also had to realize that God wanted us to face the worst—to look the possibility of death in the eye."

STAGES OF GRIEF

Psychiatrist and author Elizabeth Kübler-Ross is generally credited with identifying stages of grief through which those who experience significant losses go.[15] The first stage of processing grief is denial. Denial can occur on two levels. Sometimes we may not even be aware of feelings or possibilities. More commonly, we refuse to acknowledge them, or even to look at them. When someone we love has died, we frequently hear words such as

"It can't be, I just saw her the other day."
"He and I were talking on the phone just hours ago."
"We had lunch last week."
"He looked to be in the best of health."

When death is imminent from a chronic disease such as cancer, denial is often present as well. Like Casey and Debbie, even when there is an awareness of what is coming, there is a reluctance to use the D word. We just don't like to think about death. Yet death is a reality. And grief is its essential attendant.

Perhaps denial was a part of David's mind-set on the day his son Absalom was killed by David's commander Joab. Sitting in his place of authority in the city gate of Jerusalem awaiting word of the battle, the primary thought in the king's mind was voiced in his initial question to the Cushite messenger who arrived to deliver the news of victory: "Is the young man Absalom safe?" Certainly the question, with its hoped-for positive response, left room for denial. But the messenger immediately shattered any denial David felt. "May the enemies of my lord the king, and all who rise against you to do you harm, be as that young man is!" (2 Samuel 18:32). David immediately began to experience the next stages of grief—strong emotions.

The deeper the loss
and the more unexpected the loss,
the longer it takes for grief
to be processed to resolution.

These include anger turned *inward,* perhaps because we feel guilty over the person's death or believe we might have done something to prevent it, anger turned *outward,* perhaps because not everything that could have been done medically was done, or we may simply be angry with the person who died or with others we see as somehow being to blame for the loss we have suffered. Or our anger may be focused upward, directed toward God. We may even verbalize the kind of emotion Martha expressed when she said, "Lord, if You had been here, my brother would not have died" (John 11:21).

Frequently these strong emotions fluctuate wildly, swinging back and forth like the needle of a seismograph during an earthquake. David's immediate response was to rush to his chamber over the gate, pour out his tears, and cry out, "O my son, Absalom—my son, my son, Absalom—if only I had died in your place. O Absalom, my son, my son" (2 Samuel 18:33). Intense emotions. Anger directed inward, outward, even upward, in a random, rapid-fire sequence. All of this is a common part of the grief process.

At some point in the grief process, we may even try to bargain with God. "I'll do anything for you, Lord. Just bring my loved one back," or, "Don't let my loved one die."

When does grief come to resolution? At different times and in different ways for different people. The general rule is, the deeper the loss and the more unexpected the loss, the longer it takes for grief to be processed to resolution. However, grief is generally resolved when we finally come to a point of realistic acceptance of our loss. Frequently this involves the shedding of tears. It always involves owning our painful feelings of anger, hurt, and loss.

SHOULD CHRISTIANS GRIEVE?

Two questions arise from our discussion of grief. First, can someone close to a person dying of a chronic disease such as cancer begin to grieve before the death? Second, should Christians—committed to Christ, believing in the hope of everlasting life—grieve? The answer to both these questions is yes.

In response to the second question, it is not only appropriate but normal and necessary for people of faith to grieve. David grieved deeply over the loss of Absalom. Earlier in life, he expressed his grief over the death of his infant son born to Bathsheba. Jacob mourned deeply the loss of his son Joseph, whom he thought to be dead. And Jesus wept at the tomb of Lazarus. Even though He knew He was about to restore His friend to life, He still wept.

Frequently, well-meaning people will urge believers not to mourn or even weep over the death of a loved one. Sometimes, an improper understanding of statements such as Paul's in 1 Thessalonians 4:13 contribute to the confusion. Writing words of encouragement to Christians who have experienced the death of family or close friends, Paul explains the hope of resurrection "lest you sorrow as others who have no hope." Significantly, he does *not* say that you should not have sorrow. From Paul's perspective, it was appropriate for Christians to sorrow, to grieve, even to mourn and weep over the loss of a loved one. However, the sorrow and the grief of a believer differs significantly from that of one who has no hope in Christ. The reason for this difference is simple, yet profound. For the believer, death is viewed as a temporary separation. That's why Paul uses the words "those who have fallen asleep" to describe the separation of death.

Thus, for Casey and others who mourned Debbie's passing, a primary source of comfort was the anticipation of reunion in the presence of God, in a place where there will never be tears, sorrow, suffering, separation, or death. Heaven is the ultimate encouragement for believers in the face of grief.

In many instances, anticipatory grief actually begins well before the point of death. That was David's experience when his infant child became gravely ill. Pleading with God to spare the child, David fasted and withdrew from the company of others, even refusing to eat. Grief over an anticipated loss mingled with fear of the loss. Once the child had died, David was able to bring his grief to quick resolution, resuming such daily activities as meals, fellowship, and worship. A key factor in the resolution of David's grief—which seemed to occur far more rapidly than that of most people who suffer such a loss—was the ultimate confidence David expressed: "I shall go to him, but he shall not return to me" (2 Samuel 12:23).

It is important not to place time expectations on those who grieve. Grief is an intensely personal matter. Everyone's experience of grief is different. However, it is extremely common for those facing the loss of a loved one to a chronic disease such as cancer to begin processing grief long before the actual death occurs. Even then, a year or more is a common period for grief to continue after such a severe loss.

All through those final months, Debbie and Casey kept processing their grief. "There were times we'd express our anger to each other. We'd cry out honestly to God. And we had friends we could level with." They worked through the stages, from denial to anger. At other times, they felt guilt—What if I'd done something different? What if I just changed certain things? Why me? Why us? At other times, they felt a sense of peace, believing God to have a purpose in it all.

Purpose in Death

At still other times, Debbie and Casey were convinced that somehow God was going to "pull things out of the bag," work a miracle. One such time came shortly after the hiring of a housekeeper to look after young Spencer. "We ran an ad in the local *Green Sheet* and had just one phone call in response. She had such a cheerful spirit, such great faith. I became convinced that God had sent her along to be the agent through which Debbie would be healed.

"Today, I'm sure that she, and others we know, think Debbie died because we just didn't have enough faith. Sometimes we'd pray, 'Lord, if it's Your will, let Debbie be healed.' She'd say, 'No, no. Don't pray that way. It's never God's will for anyone to be sick.'"

Looking back, Casey has been able to affirm that there are times when sickness, suffering, and even death can be God's will. Clearly it was God's will for Paul to suffer from his physical "thorn," and for Lazarus to be sick, then die. Likewise, for David's infant son.

Casey admitted, "I'd been asking 'Why,' struggling to find a purpose in all this. Then just before Debbie died, our Bible study teacher from church shared two verses with me from Isaiah 57. I had never seen them before."

The verses Casey remembered spoke vividly to the issue of death, specifically to those who die in faith: "The righteous perishes, and no man takes it to heart; merciful men are taken away, while no one considers that the righteous is taken away from evil. He shall enter into peace; they shall rest in their beds, each one walking in his uprightness" (vv. 1–2).

Casey recalled the hushed silence of the hospital corridor and the words quoted by his friend. "[He] told me that, although we can't understand God's full purpose, there were two things we could consider in facing the death of a believer like Debbie. First, she was taken away from evil. Her physical suffering, her continued ups and downs, would be over. Second, she would enter into peace and rest, going to that place every one of us who knows the Lord longs for."

After receiving those verses, Casey read them over and over, committed them to memory, then used them as a major source of support during the final thirty-six hours of Debbie's life and in the days following her death. "The comfort of Scripture—especially those verses—provided me with major support to get through this time of loss."

A second key source of support for Casey and Debbie as they processed their grief was the prayer and encouragement of Christian friends. "Our Bible study class, other classes, special individuals. My friend Duncan, the guy who discipled me, spent several nights at the hospital, sitting up with me. He was incredible. He's married, has three kids and a job—but he was just there for us. Others were too."

Earlier, Greg had fasted for three days as he prayed for Debbie's cure. Others fasted as well. Many prayed. Some held all-night prayer vigils. "There was a lot of hands-on praying," Casey explained.

During this time, Casey began to put into perspective the issue of praying and the power of God, reconciling it with the purpose and plan of God. "I don't understand all there is to know about that. Probably none of us does. Looking back now though, I can see a lot of God's purpose. He used Debbie's death in such a great way in so many lives, mine included. Even up until the very end, we didn't give up hope. There were three special friends who prayed with me regularly. If Debbie's recovery had depended on the intensity of our prayers, there would have been no question about the outcome. And while we were praying, we didn't stop trying every possible treatment resource. We believed in praying as though it all depends on God, plus doing everything we possibly could, including conventional treatments, and even experimental therapy."

Prior to her hospitalization Debbie had undergone an experimental hormonal therapy—Tamoxifen, an estrogen blocker. "They told us 30 percent of the women who take this experience up to a two-year remission. We tried two others. They didn't work either. Each time our hope was diminished."

Following the hormonal therapy, the Burke's consulted with Dr. Jones about an experimental treatment called Gemcitabine. "She had been in a lot of pain, couldn't sleep at night. The ulcerated sore in her chest just kept growing. But when they started her on this Gemcitabine treatment, the wound started healing up. She began to feel better and was able to rest. For three weeks, we were convinced this was going to cure her." It was during this time that Debbie was able to attend church for what was to be the last time.

"Then the next week we went for another checkup. Both of us were happy and positive about the progress we thought she was making." But when Dr. Jones walked into the office, the frown on his face was like a cloud dampening their mood. "It just isn't working," he told them. As both Debbie and Casey began to protest, he pointed to the edges of Debbie's surgical scar. "Feel these," he said, indicating a series of bumps or small knots. "They wouldn't be there if it were working."

Casey recalled their feelings as they left the doctor's office after that visit: "It was like we had been run over by a truck—again."

Debbie and Casey were so desperate they ever tried one of the countless theories outside the medical community. "We had heard about all the different things people recommend: fruit juice therapies, coffee enemas, the Chinese doctor who gives you two pills and you're cured. It seemed we read thousands of books. Things like *Love Medicine and Miracles,* about people *thinking* themselves well. We heard of this guy in Michigan who made some stuff that supposedly caused the cancer cells to kill themselves. I ordered some, and Debbie took it. It was horrible tasting. But it didn't work."

Death is something we don't like to talk about.

Random memories stood out to Casey as he thought about those final two weeks Debbie spent in Baylor Hospital before her death in mid-July 1991. "My friend Greg and I wheeled Debbie into a room across the hall and held her up so she could see the Fourth of July fireworks at the Cotton Bowl. The guy who had been in that room had died that morning. Watching the fireworks was a fun event. But my most vivid memory was when we held Debbie up to watch. Wherever we pressed on her to support her, our fingers would leave deep impressions in her skin. She was extremely swollen, since her liver and kidneys weren't working. Even though we enjoyed the fireworks, I felt very sad.

"Earlier that day, Debbie had seen her son, Spencer, twice. The last time he kissed her hand. She reached out to him, and he said, 'Good night, Mommy. Hope you feel better.' Then he and I went out and picnicked by the fountain. He made a wish for his mommy on his own!"

The next day, Debbie told Casey that it had really hit her that she wasn't going to leave the hospital. She found it increasingly hard to breathe. A few days later, as she struggled to stay awake because of the pain medication, Debbie talked with Casey at length about what lay ahead. "We talked about how, if she didn't come home, she knew she would be with Jesus. Then she gave me a hug. That afternoon she lost consciousness for good. She died at 8:25 the following evening."

Preparing for Death

Death is something we don't like to talk about. We frequently use words like "departed" or "passed away" to lessen the impact. But each of us has an appointment with death. Statistically, more people die of cardiovascular disease. Cancer ranks as the second-leading cause of death. Accidents, pulmonary disease, diabetes, even homicide are also listed among the other leading causes of death. Death is a certainty for every human being.

Perhaps the greatest difference between cancer and other causes of death, such as cardiovascular disease, accidents, or homicide, is that cancer often gives the patient and the family time to prepare. So how can those who are dying with cancer and those who are close to them prepare?

First, *set aside denial.* It is important to recognize that denial is a normal, common human defense mechanism. But denial of impending death is no more constructive than denying the reality of the April 15 deadline for federal income taxes or the existence of a toothache-causing cavity. Facing the possibility, even the likelihood, of death—without denial and without giving up hope—is essential.

Second, even in the face of death, *don't give up hope.* Continue to pursue both prayer and all the appropriate treatment options. This balanced approach, referred to elsewhere in this book as *active waiting,* is an especially important coping tool. It doesn't deny the reality of hope or the possibility of divine intervention, but it recognizes the balanced truth expressed by Paul that "to live is Christ, and to die is gain" (Phillipians 1:21).

Third, *don't be ashamed to express, share, and process emotions.* Since cancer is chronic, grief will precede the actual death. Grief can be expected both before and after death occurs. Processing those intense emotions, rather than burying them, is the most healthy approach.

Fourth, *set your house in order.* Those were the words used by Isaiah the prophet in warning Israel's King Hezekiah of his impending death (Isaiah 38:1). Those were the same words quoted by Henry, a successful businessman in his late forties, when his pastor stopped to visit the night before he was to undergo a serious operation. When asked about the papers he had scattered across the bed before him, Henry replied, "I'm setting my house in order, getting ready to face death."

Ironically, Henry did not survive the next day's operation. The point of Henry's story is not to raise the issue of death premonitions, but to highlight the importance of preparing for both contingencies: life *and* death. Such preparation includes drawing up a will, making sure significant others (such as spouse and children) know the location of important papers, and making sure funeral and burial arrangements and wishes are communicated. Casey recalled that "Debbie had taken care of all that. Since she was a lawyer, she believed in having your will and all those things taken care of."

Such preparation also includes wrestling with the degree to which heroic measures will be used to prolong life. Many questions have been raised as modern technology encounters the reality of death. It is important for family members and physicians to discuss the level at which medical intervention will continue. Recent laws have been passed in many states to permit individuals to leave written instructions for family and physicians that, whenever illness makes it impossible for them to express their wishes or makes recovery unlikely, they do not wish to permit or undergo extraordinary measures to prolong life.

This seems to provide a middle-ground approach to a thorny issue that, on the one hand, could deteriorate to physician-assisted suicide and, on the other hand, could prolong a semblance of life long after a patient is actually brain dead. *We strongly encourage those who are facing this trauma to talk candidly with their physician, pastor, and spouse or close family members in order to establish and communicate precisely where the patient desires the line regarding that level of care to be drawn.*

A word to physicians at this point: Straightforward honesty regarding the diagnosis and realistic communication of the prognosis from physician to patient and family is essential. While many physicians may find it extremely uncomfortable to communicate candidly with a patient whose prognosis may be extremely poor, it is essential nonetheless. It is also helpful for the physician to communicate with the patient and the immediate family at the same time, if at all possible. This way everyone knows at the same time, and everyone knows what the others know. Such a discussion may be unpleasant, but in our opinion it is essential.

Such action on the part of a physician can help the patient follow our next suggestion. *Confront your fears and express your feelings about death.* Although such feelings and fears will vary from person to person, the fear of death is a common human experience—the source of a lifetime of bondage (Hebrews 2:15).

Yet the truth of the death and resurrection of Jesus Christ (Hebrews 2:9, 14) and the personal encouragement of Christ (Hebrews 2:18) and of God's people (3:13) can make it possible for us to face that fear honestly and confidently.

Veda had been told that she would die of cancer years before. In response to a question from her young pastor, she replied, "'Sure, I'm afraid of dying. I think everyone is.' But I finally came to the place where I could admit I was afraid. I learned to talk to my husband and some close friends about my feelings and my fears. I can't tell you what a difference that made."

For Casey and Debbie, the loving, supportive climate of friends, family, pastor, and other believers provided an atmosphere in which those fears and feelings could be faced and processed.

Finally, *look for meaning, even in death.* This can only happen when we have taken significant steps to process our feelings about death, when we have honestly faced such common questions as,

"Why did this happen?"
"Why me?"
"What terrible thing have I done?"
"Why now, just when she was in the prime of life? Why such a loving mother and dedicated Christian? Why would God let her have cancer?"

When we honestly face the "why" questions and admit that we do not have answers, we can look beyond the "why" to the "what." Job came to this point as he processed his emotions about his losses, including the deaths of his seven sons and three daughters. "I'm going through a trying time," he was able to acknowledge. "But God hasn't abandoned me. He will see to it that ultimately, good comes even from this evil. I will be refined like gold" (see Job 23:10).

Meaning in Death

It isn't always easy to search for meaning in the midst of the losses of death. But it is possible, both for the patient and the family.

Vernon had been diagnosed with leukemia at age forty-two. A hard-working executive, on his way up the ladder of success, his emotions initially ranged from rage to fear. Finally, after processing those feelings, he was able to say, "I can't believe the good things that have happened to me. I found out how much my wife loves me and how deeply I love her. Lying in this hospital bed day after day, facing what amounts to a death sentence, I've been forced to reexamine my values. I worked so hard for things—prestige, success—now my *relationships* are far more important—my wife, my children, my friends from church.

"Most of all, I've drawn closer to God. Oh, I've had plenty of times when I unloaded my anger on Him. But I've grown closer to Him than I've ever been in life, and I know I'll be even closer after I die. There's another factor too. I know of several people who have been open to listen to me or to others tell them about Christ. I never had time to witness before I was diagnosed with cancer. Now I already know of at least one person our pastor has led to Christ out of a discussion about my sickness. Maybe others will come to Him as well."

Finding meaning in Debbie's sickness and death was a key part of how Casey coped with the loss of his wife. "God worked in so many ways. I know of at least two individuals who came to personal faith through her testimony and her death. I couldn't begin to count the individuals who were challenged to pray, to trust God, and to rest in the reality of His grace in the face of pain and adversity."

When Veda finally lost her ten-year battle with cancer, her funeral, like Debbie's, provided a positive opportunity to present the good news of Christ, the hope of life beyond death.

At least three people were led to Christ immediately after her funeral. One, a brother, knelt in the cemetery with the young pastor who conducted the service and prayed to receive the Savior in whom his sister had trusted.

"Debbie and I talked about it," Casey recalled. "Several times before her death, she expressed—and I did too—how we wanted God to use all this for His glory. He certainly did so. And He provided for all our needs. He took care of our son, Spencer, and me in ways I couldn't even imagine."

Surrounded by close friends even after his loss, Casey was able to continue to process the grief he felt over losing Debbie. Then, several months later, God brought a young, single lady into his life. Her name was Andrea.

"I figured it would be at least a couple of years before I even thought about remarriage, much less entertained the idea. Andrea wasn't looking to get married either. She was happily single and successful in her career. But she was godly—attractive, too. Our friendship developed, and God really used her to help me process a lot of my grief over losing Debbie. We spent so much time just talking together, sharing feelings. Andrea is a wonderful listener. She helped me get feelings out I didn't even know I had. I think being able to share those kinds of deep feelings with her helped draw us closer together than would normally be possible in a matter of months."

Today Casey is married to Andrea, raising the son God gave him and Debbie. He and Andrea are expecting a new child. "I don't want to kid anybody. I lived with cancer, and the person who was closer to me than anybody died of it. I can't think of many things that could be harder. But through it all, I really saw how good God is. It's like that poem and the picture about the footprints in the sand. Sometimes I felt abandoned by God, but now I know that when there was just one set of footprints, He carried me through."

11

PREVENTING CANCER

Puffy, summerlike clouds punctuated the sunshine on a warmer than usual February day as the family cancer support group gathered at Betty and Robert's home for a special birthday celebration. It was Sunday afternoon, Valentine's Day. Jimmy, Betty's older brother, would celebrate his seventy-fifth birthday the next day. Two days later Betty would turn sixty-six.

The glassed-in porch, with its comfortable furniture and view of the combination of evergreens and hardwoods behind the Norton home, gave an illusion of warmth to what was a sunny but still brisk February afternoon. Betty had prepared a special birthday meal and ordered a strawberry cheesecake from a nearby German bakery in honor of the birthday celebration.

As Betty and Robert, Jimmy and his wife, Juanita, their sister Carolyn, and sisters-in-law Jean and Bea gathered on the porch, the conversation ranged from the unusually mild February weather to the fact that Robert had obviously tilled his garden plot in preparation for planting, which, as he told everyone, was "just around the corner."

"We meet regularly as a family cancer support group," Betty explained. "But we rarely talk about cancer. We just get together to encourage each other. We started this when Dorothy, our oldest sister, was diagnosed with colon cancer back in '86. We've been meeting every couple of months or so, just to encourage each other, for about seven years now."

A Cancer-Plagued Family

Perhaps it seems unusual that Betty and Jimmy and their spouses and relatives would meet regularly as a family cancer support group. However, as Betty, a retired high school librarian and acknowledged family historian, noted, "Cancer and our family have been connected in some way or another ever since my parents were fairly young, when my mother's sister died of breast cancer. Her son—our first cousin—died of lung cancer when he was in his forties. Then our oldest brother, Stanley, lost his first-born son David—my parents' first grandson—to a malignant brain tumor back in 1943."

Earlier that day Betty's voice had cracked with emotion as she explained how the family in which she and Jim were raised had been decimated by cancer. "'76, '79, '80, '86, '89, and '90— those were years Jimmy and I lost a brother or a sister to cancer. And each one had a different kind. Stanley died of cancer of the pancreas in '76. We lost Bill to lung cancer in '79. The next year Ruth died of breast cancer. Then Margie died of bladder cancer in '86. Don died of prostate cancer in '89. Then we lost Dorothy to colon cancer in '90. It almost seems like our family must have set some kind of record."

It is indeed an incredible record. Four brothers and two sisters, all dead from cancer over a fourteen-year period, and each from a different form of cancer. In addition, Carolyn, the surviving sister, had a kidney removed because of cancer in 1982. Then Jeff, another brother, underwent surgery for prostate cancer in 1992.

It is not surprising that giving each other emotional and spiritual support for cancer would be a priority for Betty and Jimmy's family—or that cancer prevention would be near the top of Betty's personal priority list. And Jimmy's.

With a youthful energy belying his seventy-five years, a slim 173 pounds on his just-under-six-foot frame, a full head of silver-gray hair and piercing blue eyes, Jimmy sat back, crossed his legs, and stroked his chin thoughtfully. "He has a stomach as flat as a thirty-year-old—exercising, swimming, walking, eating right, all that keeps him in such good shape," his wife, Juanita, explained.

Jimmy took a sip of coffee. "There were twelve of us kids in the family altogether. Two died in childhood. Betty and I are the only surviving members of the family who haven't been diagnosed with cancer. Two others, Jeff and Carolyn, have survived major cancer surgery. So six of us have died from one form of cancer or another since 1976. I don't think it would take a genius to figure out why Betty and I both make cancer prevention a priority."

Cancer Prevention

Some people still don't believe that cancer can be prevented. However, as earlier chapters in this book have indicated, when it comes to cancer, Ben Franklin was right: an ounce of prevention can certainly be worth a pound of cure.

Whether a person has been diagnosed with it in the past or not, cancer prevention is a subject of major importance. For those who have never had cancer, it is possible to take certain steps to help keep the disease from occurring. For those who have already been diagnosed with cancer, whether still in the process of treatment or beyond the point of being declared "cancer free," preventing cancer's recurrence can be a virtual lifesaver.

Dr. Mark Renneker, assistant clinical professor in the department of Family and Community Medicine at the University of California San Francisco, has practiced at the Cancer Education and Prevention Center in Oakland and has served as a member of the board of directors of the California division of the American Cancer Society. He tells a story he heard in medical school that puts cancer prevention into perspective:

> A physician described himself as standing by the shore of a swiftly flowing river. Hearing the cry of a drowning man, he leaps into the river, pulls the man to shore and applies artificial respiration. Just as the near-drowning victim begins to breathe, the physician hears another cry for help. So he jumps into the river, pulls a second drowning victim to shore and again gives artificial respiration. Just as that victim begins to cough, sputter and breathe, there is yet another cry for help. Again and again the sequence continues.

Suddenly it dawns on the doctor that he is so busy jumping in, pulling victims to shore and giving artificial respiration, that he has no time to go upstream to find out and stop whoever or whatever is pushing them into the water in the first place.[1]

Today, despite the fact that some people don't believe cancer can be prevented, a great deal of money and time is being spent trying to prevent cancer. One cancer prevention skeptic was Liz (story in chapters 2, 7), who was quick to voice her doubts during an appointment at which Dr. Franklin, her family physician, had been encouraging her husband to have a checkup and take other steps to remain cancer free.

"I just don't believe you can prevent cancer, Dr. Franklin. After all, what's the point? My mother died of stomach cancer. My daughter had to have a mastectomy. Now I've had cancer. I mean, you're either gonna get it, or you'll avoid it."

Dr. Franklin shook his head in disagreement. "Liz, I can certainly understand your feelings. But I suspect you're like a lot of people—particularly those who have been diagnosed with cancer. Let me explain cancer prevention in a way that may shed some light on the subject and encourage both you and Bill to practice cancer prevention."

Picking up a blue marker, Dr. Franklin erased the notes left over from a previous session, then wrote the words "Primary Prevention" across the top of the acrylic board in his office. "When we're talking about primary prevention, we're talking about the *absence* of disease. In other words, no cancer at all. It's sort of like. . . . When you and Bill were children, you were probably vaccinated for polio, weren't you?"

Bill and Liz both nodded. "Salk vaccine, right?" Liz countered. "Or Sabin. But what does that have to do with cancer? Polio vaccine kept us from getting polio, not cancer."

"Point well taken," Dr. Franklin patiently responded. "What I'm getting at is, just as your parents took the step to have you vaccinated against polio, there are steps that you can take at a primary level to keep from getting cancer. Unfortunately, when it comes to cancer, there are still a lot of people today who take the same approach that they take with their automobile. They wait until it breaks before fixing it."

"What you are saying makes sense," Bill observed. "I've always been strong on preventive maintenance for my car—

changing the oil on time, breaking in an engine carefully whenever I purchase a new car, getting tune-ups, having the brake linings checked. I've found it's a good way to keep from being left by the side of the road."

"That's precisely what I'm talking about. But the line between *primary* and *secondary* prevention is sometimes hard to tell. Secondary prevention is the major thrust of cancer prevention today." Dr. Franklin wrote the words "Secondary Prevention" on the board under the first line of writing, then underlined the two words he had written.

"Let me explain why secondary prevention is so crucial." Pausing, Dr. Franklin picked up another marker from the tray— a red one—then wrote the words "Asymptomatic Disease."

"So what is *asymptomatic disease?*" Liz asked, shifting to the edge of her chair. "Is there a kind of cancer that doesn't have any symptoms?"

"Not exactly, Liz. *Asymptomatic* means that the disease is present, but it isn't causing any recognizable symptoms. In the past, it seems that all our efforts at cancer education were focused on detecting the earliest symptoms or *warning signs* of cancer—and they're still important. But by the time noticeable symptoms begin to appear, the chance of curing the cancer is already significantly lower than if it's caught earlier. Let me explain."

Erasing the words he had written on his marker board, Dr. Franklin drew a black circle, placing a small black dot in the middle of it. To the side he drew a triangle in red. With the red marker he drew an arrow from the triangle to the black dot inside the circle. Then he turned to face Liz and Bill.

"Imagine that this is a normal cell," he said, pointing to the circle with the black dot in the middle. Then he pointed to the triangle. "And this is a carcinogen, a cancer-causing agent. As you've already learned, cancer-causing agents bombard the cells in our bodies all the time. There's a good chance cancer cells form over and over in the bodies of most healthy people, only to be killed by the body's natural defenses."

Drawing a square around the shapes he had placed at the top of his marker board, Dr. Franklin then wrote the words "Primary Prevention" in blue to the side of the box.

Beneath the first box he drew a second, larger box and labeled it "Secondary Prevention." Bill and Liz watched as he drew two black circles inside the second box. He then drew lines from the circle in the first box to connect with the two circles at the top of the second box. Picking up the red marker, he placed a red dot inside the two circles.

"This is where secondary prevention begins—where screening and early detection is crucial—like getting a Pap test to find cervical cancer or having a digital exam to discover any signs of prostate cancer."

Dr. Franklin wrote the words "cancer cells" between the two circles in the second box, the ones with the red dots in the middle. "This represents the first doubling of malignant cells. This is what cancer cells do in the human body."

Underneath each of the two circles he labeled cancer cells, the doctor formed two additional circles, spreading them across the marker board. He placed red dots inside each of these also. "These four circles represent the cells from the second doubling of malignant cells. It's easy to see the process on a board like this, but we're still a long way from any size that could possibly be detected."

As Liz and Bill continued to watch, Dr. Franklin drew two additional circles under each of the four circles on the second line, eight new cells. "What you can see now is the third doubling. That's about as far as I can show you at scale. But by the time a tumor gets to its twentieth doubling, it may contain a million cancer cells. Normally, this happens years after the carcinogen first caused the cancer. But the natural progress of cancer is that it continues to grow, multiplying by dividing, until it eventually kills the host body."

"I guess I never thought of cancer that way," Bill replied. "I sort of pictured cancer as growing explosively. Like kudzu vines. I was raised in the South where kudzu was brought in years ago to keep down erosion on graded highway slopes. Unfortunately, the kudzu vines grew so explosively they took over everything. But it sounds like what you're describing happens a lot slower."

"Well, yes and no," Dr. Franklin replied, running his hand through his thick head of white hair. "Actually a cancer cell may turn into two cells even more slowly than a normal cell. For example, a normal cell inside the colon may take three hundred days to double, while a cancerous colon cell may take as many as six hundred days before it doubles. By the time the original cancer cell has doubled twenty times, you would have a tumor with approximately a million cells. It could have taken over thirty years to grow to that size."

"That sounds pretty big, Doc," Liz injected. "Is that about the size it takes to kill you?"

"Actually, a one-million-cell cancer would probably be less than one-sixteenth of an inch across. I doubt if you could spot a tumor that size, even it were growing on the tip of your nose."

---

*That's why early screening—
regular self-examination for both
women and men—is extremely crucial.*

Returning to his marker board, Dr. Franklin placed a small red dot below the circles and squares he had drawn. It was almost impossible to see. Beside it he wrote the words "One mm tumor—20 doublings, one million cells."

"Now this little guy, even though you couldn't see him, is already a millimeter in size. But let's suppose this cancer were growing a little bit faster. Let's suppose it had doubled *thirty* times." Placing a larger red dot on the board, Dr. Franklin labeled it "One cm tumor—30 doublings, one billion cells."

"This cancer would be about a third of an inch in width. At this size it's beginning to show symptoms. But this is the point where what has seemed to be very slow growth suddenly becomes more like an avalanche." Dr. Franklin drew a third box. Inside this box, he sketched a large circle in red. It was almost as big as the box. Inside the red circle he wrote "One kg tumor—2.2 pounds, 40 doublings, one trillion cells."

"By the time the cancer gets this big, you're past the point of trouble. A tumor this size, weighing over two pounds, would probably result in death. That's why prevention is so important. You see, all these years can pass before the tumor ever reaches one centimeter in size. But between that point and the one-kilogram-size tumor—the deadly size—you have a relatively small window of opportunity to treat the cancer. By the way, treatment for an existing cancer with symptoms is what we call *tertiary prevention.*"

Dr. Franklin used the red marker to point to the third box he had drawn on the board, with the large red circle inside. "Tertiary prevention includes any cancer growth in the detectable range—from just larger than the one-centimeter size on up. It's where things are for you right now, Liz. With Bill, we hope we're still at primary prevention. But we *could* be at secondary. It's really impossible at this stage for us to tell the difference between a person who is cancer free and someone who may have the early stages of cancer growing undetected. And waiting until obvious warning signs crop up is just too big a risk to take. That's why early screening—regular self-examination for both women and men—is extremely crucial. Regular medical checkups also fall into the category of secondary cancer prevention."

"So what exactly do you consider to be primary prevention, Doc?" Bill asked.

"Things like eliminating tobacco, eating the right kinds of foods, minimizing any environmental or occupational exposure to cancer-causing agents. A lot of it is just common sense. But remember, it's your life."

Primary Prevention

Both Betty and her brother Jimmy had come to believe strongly in primary and secondary cancer prevention. Both had witnessed firsthand the grim battles that took place at the tertiary prevention level, when their brothers and sisters were treated. Carolyn, sitting next to Jimmy on the porch, recounted her fight with kidney cancer.

"It was '82. I remember the year like it was yesterday. We have a family history of diabetes, and I had just discovered that I was diabetic. I also had a heart attack that year. It must be some kind of medical feat, having cancer surgery and a heart attack all in the same year. I can laugh about it now, but it sure wasn't funny then. I was a heavy smoker up to that point. That year I quit—cold turkey."

"Primary prevention," Bea, Carolyn's sister-in-law, added. "I just wish Bill had quit. He was a pharmacist and a heavy smoker. I'm sure that was a big factor in his lung cancer. He was diagnosed in January of '79. He died June fifteenth that year, just three weeks before his fiftieth birthday."

Like Bea, Jean had lost her husband, Don, to cancer. "He and Jimmy had been in the marines during World War II. They were both strong and robust." The head of a large and successful automobile parts business, Don had seen his doctor regularly because of a juvenile onset of diabetes. He had also exercised regularly—swimming several laps in his pool almost every day.

"We had been to Hawaii that summer," Jean recalled. "Don felt really good. But on the flight back home, he began having severe back pain. He thought it was from some exercise, windsurfing or skiing, or even from sleeping on a different pillow. When the pain didn't go away, I finally convinced him to go for a checkup. By the time they found the cancer, it had spread from the prostate into the bone."

For Betty and her husband, Robert, for Jimmy and his wife, Juanita, cancer had hit extremely close to home. "None of us realized it at the time when David, our brother Stanley's oldest son, died in surgery for a brain tumor. We didn't know what a foreshadowing of things to come that would turn out to be."

Jimmy began elaborating on the losses Betty had listed earlier. "Stanley in '76. He had retired in March after his sixty-fifth birthday. He didn't feel very well. I think that's why he went ahead and retired. He had planned to keep on working—he really enjoyed his job. That summer he was diagnosed with cancer of the pancreas. He died in October."

"We lost Bill in '79," Betty picked up the story. Bea nodded as Betty continued. "He was diagnosed in January—died five months later. Like Bea said, just before his fiftieth birthday.

"I remember being there when he died," Betty recalled, shaking her head as if to deny her words. "I came to sit with Bill that night at the hospital."

"We were all just totally exhausted," Bea said. "I was in hopes that maybe Bill was taking a turn for the better. Betty offered to sit up that night, to give me a chance to get some rest."

As Bea paused, Betty continued. "I sat there all that night. Because of the damage to his lungs, Bill's breathing was extremely loud and labored. About five that morning, I realized everything was quiet. When I understood what had happened, I felt like a horse had galloped through the door and kicked me in the stomach."

When the medical staff confirmed that Bill had died, Betty couldn't even remember the phone number to call Bea and let her know. "I knew that number as well as my own. But I was in such a state of shock, I couldn't for the life of me remember it. I had to have someone look it up. I was just numb."

"Bill was the second one we lost," Jimmy continued. "Then Ruth the next year. She beat cancer for fifteen years. They first diagnosed her with breast cancer in '65. She had a radical mastectomy. Lived well beyond the five-year point when you're considered to be recovered."

"But when that kind of cancer recurs, they say it's pretty grim," Betty added. "We lost Ruth in the fall of '80, right around Thanksgiving. I remember people from her church bringing in Thanksgiving food for the family."

"After that, we went six years without losing anybody else," Jimmy recalled. "Although we had quite a scare with Carolyn's bout with kidney cancer in '82. Then we lost our sister Margie in '86. She had bladder cancer. I remember she died the day before the space shuttle exploded. She was seventy-one."

Betty picked up the story. "Then we lost Don to prostate cancer in '89. I was there when he died too."

Jean continued the narrative. "Our son and his wife brought our only grandson by that day. They were taking him to the state fair. Betty came by to sit with Don and me."

"He had been so talkative all that day," Jean remembered. "We had even discussed his faith—how he was ready to go be with the Lord but that he'd sure miss us. It seemed like he was doing pretty well. About half an hour later, it was like he just suddenly started the process of dying. It didn't take long."

Betty smiled as she paused to wipe a tear that had formed in the corner of her eye. "A lot of losses we've had."

"This family's had to have a lot of courage." Jean picked up the conversation. "I remember how strong Don's faith had become—especially near the end, when he realized what he was up against. I think both of us received a lot of support from the family. And we sensed how close the Lord was to us during that time."

"Don died in October of '89," Betty said. "Then we lost Dorothy to colon cancer in May of the next year. She died the same day as Sammy Davis, Jr., and Jim Hensen of the Muppets —all from cancer. They even printed her obituary in *USA Today*.

She had been a social worker and worked at the tumor registry at the University of Alabama Birmingham."

"The most remarkable thing about Dorothy," Jean interjected, "was how she came to faith. She had been an atheist almost her entire life—made no bones about it. But I think she saw the reality of faith in everybody else in the family. She felt a lot of love and support, even when she was going through the worst of times, during her last months."

"It was Mother's Day, just a few days before she died," Betty remembered. "Jimmy and his oldest son went to visit her in the hospital. They wanted to talk to her about the Lord one more time. They knew she had just days to live, perhaps even hours. That afternoon she trusted Christ. Three days later she was with the Lord."

"I still remember the change in her voice and the look on her face when she told me about it," Jean recalled. "We had all prayed for her for the longest time. I guess she's living proof that while there's life there's still hope."

"There's one more chapter to this cancer story," Jimmy added. "Our brother Jeff was diagnosed with prostate cancer in '91, the year after Dorothy died. He had surgery in January of '92. He's on a cancer prevention program, as you might expect. He called the other day from Atlanta, where they live. He had just had his annual exam. Said his PSA level was zero. That's great news."

Recent research has indicated that garlic . . . can play a significant role in cancer prevention.

Everyone nodded, then Robert spoke quietly from his seat next to Betty. "We're just trying to keep Betty and Jimmy from writing any more chapters in the saga of this family."

Juanita touched her husband's arm. "That's why Jimmy has been so careful to follow his own personal cancer prevention plan. It started when he quit smoking back in '57. Before that he stopped drinking alcohol of any kind in '52. Over the past few years, he and I have made an agreement to try to eat the right foods—avoid fats, cut down on red meat, and eat plenty of vegetables and fruits."

"Robert and I have followed the same plan you and Jimmy have," Betty smiled at Juanita. "And we both started making sure we went to the doctor for our annual checkup. My next one is scheduled for this coming week—I'll fast for fourteen hours, then go in for the works—mammography, the whole nine yards. Last checkup, I had no symptoms whatever."

"I started going for annual exams back in '84," Jim remembered. "I had a little prostate swelling at the time. My doctor convinced me that I needed to come in every year for a thorough checkup. I don't regret it a bit."

Cancer and Diet

In recent years, Americans have literally been bombarded with information—and sometimes misinformation—about the connection between diet and diseases like cancer. An avalanche of reports and studies has been successful in motivating many people toward a healthier diet—less red meat and animal fat, less or no alcohol, more fresh fruits and vegetables, and whole grains.

At the same time, there have been reports and books published that exaggerated claims about the benefits of certain dietary supplements. When we talk about cancer prevention, we recommend a careful analysis to distinguish between what has been established by research as *certain,* what is merely *suspected,* and what remains a *mystery.*

In the category of the certain, fat—particularly animal fat—has been implicated as a major factor in causing three of the most common types of cancer in the developed world: colon, breast, and prostate cancers. These cancers took the lives of three of Jimmy's and Betty's siblings. That's one of the main reasons they and their spouses started exercising such care to reduce their fat consumption. Being overweight is another proven risk factor. Unlike several of their brothers and sisters, both Jimmy and Betty have managed to guard against becoming overweight.

On the positive side, an increased intake of dietary fiber has been shown to lessen the risk of colorectal cancer. Eating high fiber foods from the cabbage family (such as broccoli, cauliflower, brussels sprouts, and cabbages), plus whole grains, wheat and bran cereals, potatoes, spinach, tomatoes, whole wheat bread, and other high fiber foods can contribute to general wellness and help guard against colorectal and breast cancer.

Recent research has indicated that garlic, which for thousands of years has been considered a factor in both the treatment and prevention of disease, can play a significant role in cancer prevention. Dr. Michael Wargowich, cancer researcher at M.D. Anderson Hospital in Houston, describes research into the effects of garlic on cancer prevention as "no longer nutritional-food-store stuff." Wargowich has reported significant success in using garlic compounds to prevent cancer of the stomach and esophagus in rats, and he and other researchers see important implications for preventing cancer in humans. "At our hospital [M.D. Anderson], two cancer research sections, gastrointestinal and head and neck, have committed themselves to chemopreventive studies. We realize that [garlic] presents a roadblock to a lot of tumors, and a lot of specialists in early cancers now consider this the way to go. It's really exciting."[2]

The therapeutic use of garlic dates back as far as ancient Egypt, to the sixteenth century before Christ. Aristotle, Hippocrates, and Louis Pasteur are among those who have touted garlic for its therapeutic value. However, until recent years, the virtues of garlic have been mainly ignored by Western medical authorities, lumped into the category of herbal medicine myth. Yet respected authorities such as Wargowich and Dr. Herbert Pierson, a toxicologist who until recently headed the National Cancer Institute's "designer foods" campaign to attack cancer through diet, have labeled garlic as a "veritable pharmacopoeia" of medical benefits—including cancer inhibition. Pierson stated that "the prostaglandins that stimulate cell division are the bad guys in our bodies. What garlic and onions do is alter the way that prostaglandins are made so they don't get out of control, causing runaway cell division."[3]

Wargowich has identified several substances in garlic that seem to prevent tumors. Human trials are slated to start soon, first to determine if garlic extracts produce serious side effects. Other natural food substances, including limonoids, the flavor component of oranges and other citrus fruits, are being studied to confirm what appears to be a significant benefit in preventing breast tumors. Wargowich is quick to point out, "We use more garlic at home now ... but ... it won't be a single substance that provides immunity from all cancers. It will be a blend of active agents. So we also eat lots of fruits and vegetables and fiber."[4]

A word of caution: Experts consider it a mistake to rely on any special diet as the sole means of either preventing or treating cancer. A 1991 update to published diet guidelines from the American Cancer Society summed up its dietary advice in two words: variety and moderation. For Betty and Jimmy, variety and moderation have become watchwords, not only for diet but for a total approach to life.

Without question, ours is a society in which eating so-called "junk foods" or food items composed of a lot of artificial or synthetic substances has long been the norm. Ironically, while government agencies require pet foods to contain enough basic nutrients to sustain the life of the pet, this same standard is not required of all foods sold for human consumption.

Biblical Basis for Prevention

Believe it or not, there is a biblical basis for preventing cancer. It can be summed up in one word: stewardship. Writing to Christians living in the degenerating society of Corinth, Paul warned his readers that "your body is the temple of the Holy Spirit. ... Therefore glorify God in your body and in your spirit, which are God's" (1 Corinthians 6:19–20). Paul was addressing the specific issue of sexual immorality (vv. 16–18). As noted earlier, multiple sexual partners definitely increases the risk of certain forms of cancer.

In Paul's discussion he states an important axiom, one with great practical significance for today: "All things are lawful for me, but all things are not helpful. All things are lawful for me, but I will not be brought under the power of any" (v. 12). This axiom provides a spiritual mandate for taking physical and emotional steps toward cancer prevention: *Whereas it may be completely legal and legitimate for me to fill my body with red meat, fat, chocolate candies of all sorts, and various kinds of refined foods, it will not be helpful for my well-being. Nor is it good stewardship of the body God has given me, the body in which His spirit lives. If I am to serve Him effectively, using my body for His glory, it is essential that I take care of it.*

Ironically, Paul wrote from the personal background as master of Old Testament Israelite law, part of which was devoted to detailed regulations regarding what should or should not be eaten. Many Bible scholars have gone on record as observing that the dietary laws under which Israel lived in the Old Testament were designed to provide maximum health and wellness. Whereas Christians are not under the law of Moses, we are expected to exercise both common sense and biblical care in the stewardship of our bodies. This includes the use of substances such as alcohol or tobacco. Studies have shown that heavy alcohol intake is associated with an increased risk of cancers of the oral cavity, larynx, and esophagus. The combination of drinking and smoking increases the risk of cancer of the mouth, throat, larynx, and esophagus.

There is probably no single cancer prevention step you can take that can have as dramatic and as positive a result as to quit smoking.

Janet Sackman, who in the forties and fifties modeled for Lucky Strike and Chesterfield cigarettes in magazines and on television, lost her voice box to cancer of the larynx in 1983. Today she teaches other cancer victims who have undergone laryngectomies how to talk without a larynx and warns anyone who will listen about the dangers of the product she once helped glamorize.

"Neither Jimmy nor I smoke," Betty pointed out. "Nor do we drink alcohol. He quit. I never started."

With a chuckle, Jimmy reminded her, "I tried to get you to once—remember? We had just come back from the war, and we were driving down Third Avenue in that old roadster I had. I handed you a cigarette and asked you to light it for me. You put the cigarette in one hand, the lighter in the other, and you couldn't figure out why it wouldn't light."

Laughing, Betty nodded. "I was so ignorant about smoking that I didn't realize people had to put cigarettes into their mouths to light them. That was the only time I ever tried to light a cigarette, and I've never even put one in my mouth. Never smoked, and never plan to start."

There is probably no single cancer prevention step you can take that can have as dramatic and as positive a result as to quit smoking. Scientific research has documented positive benefits from quitting, even for those who have smoked for years. Though nicotine addiction is one of the most difficult to beat, it can be done. For a few people, quitting is easy. For most others, an agonizing, ongoing battle will be necessary. Sometimes counseling can be helpful. For others, a physician can prescribe a transdermal patch to help overcome the addiction medically. But whatever it takes, through the power of God, through personal choice, through counseling and medical help, stop smoking! You've heard it before. You'll hear it again. More than one surgeon general has determined that cigarette smoking has a direct link to a variety of cancers and is extremely hazardous to your health.

Neither Betty nor Jimmy professes to be sure about why there were so many incidences of cancer in their family. Jimmy pointed to one environmental factor. "We grew up in a home fairly close to several steel mills. Just breathing the air was like smoking a couple of packs of cigarettes a day."

Betty, the family historian, suspected hereditary factors. "After all, mother's sister died of breast cancer at an early age, and her son, my cousin, died of lung cancer. So there was cancer in mother's family. I'm still working on researching the family on both sides, to see if there were other incidences."

However, Betty and Jimmy agreed that practicing cancer prevention is more important than figuring out specifically what caused cancer in relatives. "It would be good to be able to pinpoint the cause, to say we know this is it," Betty noted. "But we really are clear on the fact that both heredity and environment can play a part."

Ten Commandments for Prevention

Cancer prevention continued to be the focus of the conversation as Dr. Franklin talked with Liz and Bill. "Let me give you my Ten Commandments for Beating Cancer," he said, handing them a printed sheet of paper. "I've adapted these from information provided by the National Cancer Institute. I hope you'll look them over carefully, and—most important—follow them scrupulously.

1 *Eat foods high in fiber and low in fat.* "Bill, I'm sure if you're like me, you enjoy those thick, juicy, marbled T-bones or rib eyes. But it's crucial for you and Liz to go for the high fiber and cut out animal fat as much as possible."

2 *Avoid tobacco in any form.* "That includes smoked, chewed, or even secondary smoke. In fact, just recently the government officially classified secondhand tobacco smoke as among the most serious cancer threats. I read in the paper last week that the EPA says infants are especially at risk—as many as 300,000 a year suffer from bronchitis, pneumonia, or other infections related to secondhand smoke. The report I read suggested that secondhand smoke may cause as many as 3,000 cases of cancer each year in nonsmokers."

"I bet the tobacco industry wasn't too happy about that report," Bill grinned.

"You hit that on the head. In fact, I read where they tried to put pressure on the EPA to delay the report, or even to dilute its findings."

"I wish they would ban smoking in more public places—like restaurants and shopping malls," Liz commented. "I noticed the sign on the front of your building—*This is a smoke-free environment: Help keep it that way.* I like that."

Dr. Franklin nodded, "So do I. Especially since I don't want to be one of the secondary-smoke statistics. But let me get on with this list—we're just about out of time."

3 *Include fresh fruit, vegetables, whole grain cereals.* "In other words, a good, healthy, fiber-filled diet."

4 *Be careful about X rays.* "Avoid them whenever they're unnecessary. Now, there's a time for a mammogram or a chest X ray. But try to avoid any unnecessary X rays."

5 *Avoid alcohol.* "I encourage people to become total abstainers. If they insist on drinking, it's imperative that they do so in moderation."

6 *Avoid overexposure to the sun.* "Be sure to wear plenty of protective clothing and use sunscreen whenever you spend extended periods outdoors. That healthy-looking tan you see

on a lot of bodies could be paving the way for skin cancer down the road."

7 *Be aware of dangers in the environment.* "Keep yourself safe on the job by using protective devices such as respirators and protective clothing."

8 *Be aware of your genes.* "Now I'm not talking about Levi's. I'm referring to incidences of cancer and the family history. Liz, I don't have to tell you about the importance of being aware of your family history of breast cancer."

9 *Get your annual physical.* "Every year. More often if your physician recommends it. Every year older we are, the more important that physical becomes. The longer I've been practicing medicine, the more careful I've become to make sure I get my own annual checkup."

10 *Practice self-examination.* "Be aware of your body, and any changes that take place—any warts, moles, or other factors. Women need to practice regular breast self-examination, and a testicular self-exam is important for men. Self-examination should also include the skin, lymph nodes, the mouth, the thyroid, vaginal and rectal area—even self-testing for blood in the stool."

Emotional and Spiritual Factors

"Even though they are not on my 'Ten Commandments' list, there are also emotional factors that can help prevent cancer," Dr. Franklin continued. "Like reducing stress, making sure you don't harbor bitterness or unresolved grudges, and cutting down on Type A behavior."

"I thought Type A was what caused heart attacks," Liz interrupted.

"It does. But Type A is a combination of what we sometimes refer to as *hurry sickness* and underlying anger. I've read quite a number of studies in which Type A behavior is identified as one of the factors that leaves us more susceptible to cancer.

"And of course, there are the spiritual factors—like practicing sexual purity. I saw another study the other day that indicated that women with multiple sexual partners are more likely to develop cervical cancer. Back in the sixties, only 9 percent of cervical cancers were found in women under thirty-five. Today that figure is up to 25 percent. Two of the biggest culprits, according to this report, were the number of sexual partners and smoking. In fact, the report said smoking more than fifteen cigarettes a day doubles a woman's risk for cervical cancer. The report also mentioned that using birth control pills can increase the risk.

"So, spiritually, we need to follow biblical guidelines for sexual behavior and practice a common sense approach for taking care of our body, since it's the temple God gave us. Well, that's about it for today," Dr. Franklin said, looking at his watch. "Liz, I sure hope I have convinced you that there are steps you can take to prevent cancer."

Liz agreed. "I think I see what you're getting at now, Dr. Franklin."

Three Factors

As Betty, Jimmy, and their family members prepared to enjoy the strawberry cheesecake in celebration of the two birthdays, one could sense an atmosphere of intense determination not to allow their family to be crushed by cancer.

"When you've seen as much cancer as we have, you sort of develop a grim determination to keep fighting it," Betty observed, "or else you give up. We've talked about this off and on for the last few years. We're convinced that there are three major factors in preventing cancer.

"One is physical and medical. I can't think of anything that would keep me—or Jimmy for that matter—from getting our regular checkups, or from following all the steps for primary and secondary cancer prevention."

As Jimmy nodded agreement, Betty continued. "Then there's the emotional factor. This family cancer support group has really helped us all. I think the battles we've fought against cancer have drawn us closer together. We've learned to accept each other, support each other."

"That's right," Jean agreed. "We really have learned to support each other. We were always a close-knit family—always scheduled a lot of family get-togethers for holidays and other special occasions. But we didn't really start supporting each other on an emotional level till after we had been through several rounds against cancer. When my husband, Don, and his sister Dorothy were both fighting cancer at the same time . . . I think that's when we really learned what it means to give each other emotional support—to be there for each other, to encourage each other to express feelings, and to allow each other to have down times."

"That's when we really became family, in the fullest sense of the word," Bea added as Carolyn, Betty, and the others nodded.

"The third factor—probably the most important—is the spiritual," Betty continued. "I think our faith in God has grown right along with our support for each other. Even though we've lost several rounds, none of us has become bitter against God. We saw Dorothy come to faith and Don's faith strengthened."

"Plus," Jimmy added, "God answered prayer for Carolyn and Jeff—she's been free of cancer now for a decade, and he's doing well after his prostate surgery. I wish he could be with us today, but I'm glad Carolyn's here. And I appreciate how Bea and Jean have given and taken support along with the rest of us and allowed their faith to grow without becoming bitter."

"Three kinds of prevention," Betty said as she stood up and began walking toward the kitchen. "Physical, emotional, and spiritual. Sounds like a good transition to strawberry cheesecake."

12

RESEARCH TOWARD ELIMINATING CANCER

Phyllis dropped her handbag, spilling its contents across the floor of Dr. Carol Richards's office as she rushed into the room. "I just can't handle the prospect of a mastectomy, radiation therapy, and chemotherapy. Going through with all that just about killed my sister. I tell you, Doctor, the treatment is worse than the cure."

Holding up her hand as if to surrender, Dr. Richards said, "Why don't you tell me more about the feelings you're having about your treatment. Let's see if we can think this through together."

"I've done a lot of thinking about it already, Dr. Richards. In fact, I've stayed awake most of two nights. You were gracious to give me this long to make a decision. I know you wanted me in the hospital for surgery by tomorrow. To be frank about it, after all Lynn has been through with her surgery and treatment—and she's eleven years younger than me—I just don't know. Besides, I just heard from my cousin about the macrobiotic diet. She told me that it cured her brother of prostate cancer. She said that one of the top doctors in a hospital somewhere out East—I believe it was Philadelphia—started using this diet to treat cancer back in the seventies. According to her, there's no point in taking radiation or having radical surgery when you can treat cancer with the right kind of diet. This doctor had surgery and other kinds of therapy, but he was cured with the macrobiotic diet. She said her brother's doctor tried to talk him out of it—that the medical profession doesn't want the public to know just how effective this kind of treatment is."

Phyllis finally paused long enough to notice Dr. Richards, chin in hand, shaking her head. "So, all right, Dr. Richards. Tell me you're against it. Tell me why. It sounded too good to be true—especially after what you told me yesterday when you gave me my diagnosis."

Dr. Richards brushed her long brown hair out of her eyes. "Phyllis, if I had a dollar for every one of the stories I've heard like that one, I could retire from medicine tomorrow. The last time I checked, there were probably fifty different kinds of unproven treatments for cancer. Everything from Laetrile to the macrobiotic diet you're talking about. You can go to Greece or Germany for treatments, to Mexico for Laetrile, or to a clinic in the Bahamas run by a zoologist who uses what he calls immuno-augmentative therapy."

Phyllis shook her head, still unconvinced. "But how can you know these kinds of treatment are not effective? Aren't some of them in the research stage? I think I saw the term *investigational treatment* in one of the brochures you gave me last night."

"Phyllis, you have a unique way of getting right to the heart of the matter." Dr. Richards smiled again. "You've already identified the two sides of a most important distinction: *investigational* treatments and *unproven* treatments. Let me explain, OK?"

When Phyllis nodded, Dr. Richards walked from behind her desk and seated herself in a chair located diagonally across from the couch on which Phyllis was sitting. "Investigational treatments are what we might call the cutting edge of treatment for cancer. There are quite a few of them, including immunotherapy, biological response modifiers, hyperthermia, and some new chemo drugs. In fact, it's almost impossible to keep up with the latest investigational treatments, they change so quickly."

She pointed to a shelf on the wall beside her filled with a variety of books with medical titles and medical journals. "Why, even my library can't keep up with everything. But there's a toll-free number for the Cancer Information Service, if you're interested in finding out the latest about what's going on in the field."

Pulling a notebook from the now thoroughly jumbled contents of her purse, Phyllis said, "Here, let me jot it down."

"It's 1-800-4-CANCER. It's actually a fairly easy number to remember. Now, I would never discourage you from calling the Cancer Information Service or getting involved in a legitimate investigational treatment. But treatments like the macrobiotic diet or Laetrile are a different animal altogether."

"What do you mean?" Phyllis asked skeptically.

"Well, investigational or experimental treatments are carried out under strict standards established by the scientific community. Usually the treatments have been found to work against tumors in animals first. Then they are tested in a first phase in humans. Phase one usually involves a small number of people. Its primary purpose is to tell whether or not the treatment is safe. Once the safety issue has been resolved, phase two tests are carried out to establish whether or not the treatment is effective. In other words, a specific treatment may take care of cancer in laboratory mice, but will it have the same positive result in humans?"

Dr. Richards paused, removed her glasses, and began polishing them with a freshly pressed white handkerchief. "The third investigational phase—before a particular therapy is adopted as a standard treatment—is designed to find out whether or not a particular treatment is better than the current standard treatment modality. And if so, under what circumstances."

"What do you mean, *modality*?" Phyllis had a puzzled look on her face.

"Sorry," Dr. Richards replied, gently shaking her head as if to chide herself. "It's another one of those twenty-five cent words we medical people always seem to be using. I guess I consider *modality* just a fancy word for treatment method or strategy. By the way, some modalities, like hyperthermia—the use of heat—have been used to treat cancer off and on for hundreds of years, with very little scientific evidence. But scientists today have developed new methods of producing and directing heat. New approaches in hyperthermia are being tested in several medical centers around the country currently, as well as at the National Cancer Institute. I understand that most of the people being treated with it are patients who have tried all the standard cancer treatments."

"But what about this macrobiotic diet?" Phyllis persisted. "Didn't you tell me yesterday that diet would play a big part in my treatment? I believe you said it would be a key factor in my recovery."

"That's one of the subtle dangers of these unproven methods of cancer treatment." Dr. Richards pulled a volume from one of the shelves next to her chair. She thumbed through the book until she located a page she had marked, then she handed it to Phyllis. "Read this."

Phyllis began reading aloud at the point where someone had taken a blue felt-tipped marker and drawn a circle around the words *macrobiotic diet*:

> The macrobiotic diet, also known as the Zen macrobiotic diet, consists mainly of cereal products such as rice. Individuals following the diet must not eat any sugar, meat or animal products, and must restrict their intake of fluids. There are many variations of the macrobiotic diet. The principle of all the diets is to recommend that liquids, usually in the form of *miso* or *tamari* broths, be used only sparingly. Meats (including poultry), dairy products, tropical or semi-tropical fruits and juices, sugar, honey or anything artificial are to be avoided. The most restrictive of these diets, not usually followed today, uses only cereals, usually in the form of brown rice. Those who recommend the diet for cancer patients believe that cancer is a toxic blood condition which has developed because of poor habits.[1]

Phyllis looked up from the page. "But what about the man who started using this diet? Wasn't he cured of prostate cancer?"

"That's what he claimed. Dr. Anthony Sattilaro was his name—he was president of Philadelphia's Methodist Hospital. I've read some of his articles. He did have prostate cancer, had been treated for it with surgery and hormone therapy. After about six weeks of standard cancer treatment, he placed himself on this macrobiotic diet. But he *continued* the hormone therapy while he was on the diet.

"He always credited his cancer cure to the diet, but most of the doctors with whom I've talked think his hormone therapy was a greater factor than the diet. Doctors at the National Cancer Institute say that about 70 percent or more of patients with prostate cancer respond to the surgery and hormone therapy Dr. Sattilaro was given. They don't agree with his opinion that the macrobiotic diet was the primary cause of his improvement.

"Turn over to the next page. There's a section there that shows how the macrobiotic diet can even be *harmful* to cancer patients. Go ahead. Read it."

> The macrobiotic diet lacks nutritional elements needed even by healthy people. It is low in many vitamins and minerals. Since milk products are excluded, getting enough calcium can be a problem. For cancer patients, there can be additional difficulties. Many are already experiencing weight loss and lack of appetite. It is common for cancer patients to feel full both during and after eating. Persons on the macrobiotic diet need to eat large amounts of food, mostly bulky foods, to obtain the number of calories required by the diet. The diet does not allow vitamin and mineral supplements.[2]

"You see, Phyllis? There are all kinds of treatments you can try. There's a clinic out in California that claims to inoculate people against a microbe they call *progenitor cryptocides*, which they say is similar to the kind of bug that causes tuberculosis and leprosy. Then there's Laetrile and hydrazine sulfate. All of these have been checked out by the National Cancer Institute. Believe me, if they had found evidence to justify putting these medicines on the market, or even conducting additional clinical trials, they would have done so."

"But don't the people who develop these medications test them?" Phyllis asked.

"They usually claim they do. But, most of the time, the amount of actual experimental evidence is very small. Test results are seldom if ever published in any reputable scientific journals. Usually they're published in popular magazines of one kind or another. Proponents of these kinds of treatment actually claim to be persecuted by organized medicine and science. But I'm convinced they're usually not published in the journals because they don't have scientifically objective evidence of effective results. The records of these unproven treatments are usually pretty skimpy—or else nonexistent. Sometimes no biopsies have been done to confirm the presence of cancer in the first place. In fact, some of these people actually refuse to do biopsies because they claim a biopsy will spread cancer, which is patently untrue.

> *Almost everyone diagnosed with cancer will likely have well-meaning friends or relatives suggest an unproven method of cancer management.*

"Another way to spot unproven treatments is when you find doctors with unusual-sounding degrees, such as N.D., Doctor of Naturopathy, or Ph.N., Philosopher of Naturopathy, or my all-time favorite, MS.D., Doctor of Metaphysics."

"But what about the doctor who first used the macrobiotic diet to treat his cancer? He did get well, didn't he?"

"Yes, he did, Phyllis," Dr. Richards replied patiently. "But remember, he also took hormone therapy."

"But I thought you said he kept getting worse after his surgery and treatment?"

"That can be explained by the fact that a positive response to treatment may not be evident until five or six weeks of hormone therapy has been given. So I think that actually provides stronger evidence for the kind of *proven* therapy I'm recommending for you than some kind of radical or unusual therapy."

Unproven Therapies

Almost everyone diagnosed with cancer will likely have well-meaning friends or relatives suggest an unproven method of cancer management. Many doctors consider such methods as much a part of the problem as cancer's capacity to kill.

Two major factors seem to spur the weedlike proliferation of these unproven remedies with their enthusiastic claims: fear and greed. Fear on the part of the cancer patient and greed on the part of many who provide the treatments, often at both great expense and significant danger to the patient.

Unfortunately, another major contributing factor in the growth of these alternative therapies is the failure on the part of many cancer treatment professionals to relate to the patient on a personal basis: "The cancer quack is the beneficiary of the overworked, the incompetent, the disinterested, the brusque professional and orthodoxy's misuse and overuse of drugs, the 'no time to listen or explain' syndrome, therapy that is often prolonged and unpleasant, the fear of mental or physical incapacity, and the 'what have I got to lose?' attitude."[3]

During Debbie's intensive treatment for breast cancer (chapter 10), she and Casey experimented with two investigational therapies: tamoxifen, an estrogen blocker, and a chemical called gemcitabine. Casey recalled hearing about many different alternative therapies. "We must have been told about hundreds of different options. Fruit juice therapy, coffee enemas, hydrogen peroxide infusions—one guy even mentioned sheep wormer. We heard the story about a Chinese doctor who had taken two pills and was completely cured. When we decided to try the gemcitabine, we had attempted just about everything, and Debbie was getting rapidly worse. We felt we didn't have anything to lose."

After six months of chemotherapy had made his life miserable, Cliff (chapters 3, 8) had also been given numerous suggestions of unproven cancer treatments. His oncologist, Dr. Short, praised him for staying with his prescribed treatment. Cliff was sitting in Dr. Short's office near the end of his course of chemotherapy.

"Let me commend you, Cliff, for resisting the temptation to try some of those novel forms of treatment some cancer patients are running to today—quite frankly, many of them border on quackery. I'd be surprised if you haven't already had well-meaning friends or family members suggest Laetrile or the macrobiotic diet. One of the main problems with these unproven methods of treatment is that they appeal to a cancer patient's desperate desire for hope. And most of the people who advocate them tend to label traditional cancer treatments as unnatural or toxic."

"But isn't chemotherapy pretty toxic? After all, you did tell me you were poisoning me, Doc," Cliff responded, smiling to let Dr. Short know he wasn't being critical.

"That's true. But the treatment options we've been using have been standard—and they were given that label only after years of controlled studies proved them relatively safe and effective. We know the risks, what the side effects are, and we can tell you and other patients the chances for success. Also, standard treatment options are usually covered by insurance, and are available in just about any facility around the country that treats cancer patients.

"The other thing to watch out for is the claim that some of these things are *natural* and don't have side effects. Laetrile, for example, is supposed to be a natural product because it's made from apricot pits. Some people estimate that as many as 75,000 Americans have tried Laetrile. But the American Cancer Society has published a booklet—here, I want you to have a copy—to give a rundown on the risks of some of these unproven treatments—things like metabolic therapy, or the macrobiotic diet. And some of those so-called metabolic therapies—enemas, colon cleansing—most people feel like they're working just because they make you miserable. But there's no real clinical evidence for them.

"And there are plenty of other treatments—there's a doctor in the Bahamas who does something called IAT, some doctors use hydrazine sulfate, and a host of others. Unfortunately, a lot of those treatments do more to cure the financial problems of their proponents than the cancer of those who are treated by them."

Cliff grinned. "I see your point, Doc: 'Don't be gullible.'"

"Especially if you wind up with a recurrence, and we have to go back to chemo or radiation. That's when you may be especially tempted to try some of these unconventional therapies. Now, I do believe in supplementing your treatment with things like a good diet and relaxation. Even prayer can't hurt. And a positive mental attitude helps. But I'll tell you something else—just thinking positively isn't going to cure your cancer either. It's not just mind over matter. Those cancer cells are killers. But I recommend a sensible diet—especially high fiber foods for someone like you, who's had colon surgery. And cutting out animal fat, plus just taking care of yourself, can help keep you healthy and minimize the risk of your cancer recurring."

Ron and Dianna Eggert (chapter 3) had also been approached by people who suggested a variety of alternative cancer treatments. "We actually had people who became offended with us because we wouldn't do some of those things," Ron recalled. "We decided we wouldn't do Laetrile, wouldn't send Jessica to Mexico.

"I remember talking with a professor I had when I was in seminary—his wife had passed away with cancer shortly before. He was a big encouragement to me. He said, 'Ron, you'll have people suggest every possible treatment: Mexico, even Greece.' When I told him we'd had everything suggested to us except Greece, he laughed and said, 'Don't bother.'"

Questions to Ask

When we are asked by patients or friends about the possibility of using unproven methods of cancer treatment, we encourage them to ask serious questions:

- ✔ What solid evidence is there that this treatment will work?
- ✔ Does it sound too good to be true?
- ✔ Has it been written up in a scientific journal?
- ✔ If not, why not?
- ✔ Will I possibly be jeopardizing my chances of overcoming cancer by using this kind of treatment?

Sometimes patients are reluctant to discuss their consideration of unproven methods with their doctor. However, frank discussion of this issue is crucial. Frequently the physician may be able to recommend some kind of investigational or experimental treatment that could produce the same—or perhaps better—results than whatever unproven treatment the patient is considering.

Another factor to consider is the cost of unproven treatments. We have discovered a wide range of costs, from relatively inexpensive to extravagantly expensive. Our most common recommendation is, use the standard, carefully approved therapies first. Even when it seems all else has failed, be careful about looking at experimental or investigational treatments.

They may simply raise false hopes while adding to the patient's financial burden. And they may actually hinder the chance of recovery.

We want to be careful to present a balanced perspective on this somewhat controversial issue. There have been many times during the history of medicine when important advances have grown from humble beginnings. We also recognize that many people who have developed alternative therapies sincerely believe in the approaches they advocate. However, we believe that the principle of accountability is best served when the proper steps for investigation by appropriate agencies—such as the American Cancer Society, the American Medical Association, the Federal Food and Drug Administration, or the National Cancer Institute—are carried out.

The National Cancer Institute has, during recent years, conducted significant research into a wide range of investigational therapies. Some of these, such as immunotherapy, have been described earlier in this book. Additional research has also come up with new methods of tried and true therapy methods, such as chemotherapy. Some tests involve using chemotherapy prior to surgery or radiotherapy, or delivering drugs directly to a limited part of the body such as the liver through the use of a portable infusion pump or even an implanted pump or catheter.

Forms of investigational treatments include particle-beam radiation therapy, neutron treatment, . . . radiation sensitizers and protectors, . . . [and] lasers.

At one point, interferon was believed to be the ultimate, dramatic new "magic cure" for cancer. As we noted earlier, interferon is a protein molecule produced by the body's immune system to help combat certain diseases that are caused by viruses, such as some forms of cancer. Scientists now know that there are many kinds of interferons. Interferon seems to be most effective with small tumors; but larger tumors have not responded well to interferon.

One recent anticancer drug approved to treat advanced ovarian cancer is a substance called taxol, which is made from the bark of the yew tree. According to Dr. Sam Broder, Director of the National Cancer Institute, taxol has produced encouraging results in many cases of advanced ovarian cancer. Current Food and Drug Administration guidelines call for it to be used in patients who have failed to respond to at least one round of chemotherapy.

Taxol was once in short supply, because its sole source was the bark of the Pacific yew tree, which is found primarily in original-growth forests protected by environmental restrictions. However, recent technological advances have allowed taxol to be made from the needles and twigs of more plentiful species of the yew tree found in Europe and Asia. There is no synthetic version of taxol. Studies have shown that taxol can shrink tumors by at least 50 percent in up to nearly one-third of women whose cancer has not responded to other therapies.[4]

Other forms of investigational treatments include particle-beam radiation therapy, neutron treatment, and even radiation sensitizers and protectors, which can make cancer cells more sensitive to radiation or chemotherapy. Lasers are frequently used to cut out or vaporize very small tumors without damaging surrounding cells. Some lasers can even be inserted into a patient's body through an endoscope and, guided by use of a fiber-optic tube, actually cut away tumors from within. Of course, any attempt at this point to comprehensively list the wide range of investigational therapies currently under development would only serve to make this book out-of-date almost as soon as it is published.

After discussion with her doctor, Phyllis finally agreed to surgery followed by a high-dose chemotherapy treatment program combined with autologous bone marrow transplants. Dr. Richards explained it to her this way: "Phyllis, we're going to use a higher dose of chemotherapy to treat you, since the higher the dosage, the more effective the treatment in killing any leftover cancer cells. But as you probably have heard, higher doses generally mean more pronounced side effects. One I'm particularly concerned about is the suppression of your immune system, which could leave you exposed to potential infections. That's why we've developed a program that's only found in a few places—one is here, another is at Spring Branch

Medical Center near Houston. We put you into a protective wing in the hospital. This protected unit has special air filters to keep the treatment environment clean and to cut down on the risk of infection."

"What about this bone marrow business? What was the word you used—autonomous?"

"Autologous," Dr. Richards replied with a grin. "It's just a way of saying that we harvest some of your own bone marrow, make sure it has been purged of any cancer cells, then reinfuse it into your body after the high-dose chemotherapy. It's the best way we've found to keep your blood count high and your infection risk low."

The National Cancer Institute works hand in hand with major cancer centers across the United States, developing investigational treatments at facilities such as the University of Texas M.D. Anderson Hospital and Tumor Institute in Houston, Memorial Sloan-Kettering in New York, the University of Alabama at Birmingham Comprehensive Cancer Center, and the Children's Cancer Research Institute at San Francisco's Pacific Presbyterian Medical Center, among many others.

Wrestling with the Options

Given the complexity of cancer, the wide variety of treatment options available, and the incredible impact cancer has on the lives of those who have it and their families, just deciding what to do can sometimes be overwhelming. *Overwhelming* was the word Candy Wood (chapter 6) used to describe her emotions when she learned her diagnosis. She faced three options: "I could have gone to the major cancer center right here in Birmingham, or to M.D. Anderson in Houston. My third option was the Mayo Clinic. I ran into my friend Dr. Raleigh Kemp, and he arranged for a biopsy to be sent there.

"That night I got down on my knees and prayed, 'OK, God. You're the only one who knows exactly what kind of tumor is in my head. You're the only one who can take care of it best. Now, I don't know how You do this, Lord. But like I told You already, I want *You* to take control. I mean, You let me know where You want me to go. I really don't know how to make this decision, Lord, and I'm afraid to depend on any person. You're the only one who knows how to do this. Now, I know You probably won't drop me a note from heaven, Lord, but whatever it takes, let me know.'

"That's how I prayed," Candy said. "And I just didn't feel peace about M.D. Anderson. So it was between UAB here in Birmingham and the Mayo Clinic. After I prayed on Friday, I was supposed to go for treatment the following Tuesday, one place or the other. That Friday evening I called Dr. Jackson, the doctor from Scotland, at the Mayo Clinic. He was to have flown in from Spain at four o'clock on Friday afternoon. It was about seven when I called his home. His wife answered the phone, and I couldn't believe it. She said he was actually there! When he came to the phone, I said, 'This is Candy Wood, Dr. Jackson. I'm really sorry for calling you on Friday night. You probably don't even know who I am . . .'

"Dr. Jackson had been in Spain for three weeks—he had just stepped off the plane a few hours before. But he says, 'Yes, Candy, I *do* know who you are. I stopped by the Mayo Clinic on my way home and ran into Raleigh Kemp. I've looked at your tomography and seen the results of your tests.'

"I knew he must be exhausted from jet lag, but he was so nice to me. And he had that Scottish accent. It just built my confidence.

"But the main thing was, I sensed he took a personal interest in me. He even took the time to describe exactly how he would perform the surgery, with an incision across the top of my head. The way he described the procedure scared me—really frightened me. When I hung up the phone, I remember praying, 'Oh, God. Please don't choose him.'

"But I kept praying about it over the weekend. And I tried to reach the doctor at UAB. For some reason, he didn't have the time that weekend to discuss the treatment with me. I'm not criticizing him for that—I'm sure he is an extremely busy physician. But it was like the Lord used those circumstances and the peace to show me, 'Candy, this is the way for you. Go to the Mayo Clinic.' I just sensed His direction."

Candy's experience again highlights that most important of principles we have sought to underscore throughout *When Cancer Comes*—combining the highest quality medical care with an active faith, waiting in dependence on the Lord.

Warfare on Three Fronts

A question we hear with a fair amount of frequency was voiced by Phyllis during the course of her talk with Dr. Richards: "Why haven't they found a cure for cancer? I mean, one cure that will just deal with the whole thing? You know, eradicate cancer completely." Since there are more than a hundred different kinds of cancer, and since cancer is a part of the breakdown in the creative process in the universe caused by sin, we believe that eradicating cancer is highly unlikely.

If cancer will continue to be a factor for the rest of human history, what are we to do about preventing it when it hasn't occurred and confronting it when it comes? There are three key areas in which cancer has an impact, three key arenas in which cancer must be confronted. These are identified in 1 Thessalonians 5:23: "May the God of peace Himself sanctify you completely; and may your whole *spirit*, *soul*, and *body* be preserved blameless at the coming of the Lord Jesus Christ" (italics added).

The ultimate key to successfully coping with cancer ... comes from the resources we receive from God when we trust His Son as our Savior.

Throughout the book we have noted that cancer has physical, emotional, and spiritual implications. As we conclude our consideration of this dreaded disease, a view of the appropriate strategies for mobilizing our physical, emotional, and spiritual resources against cancer seems in order. Although we usually begin by considering the physical, Paul starts his discussion with the spiritual, making it the priority issue. His order—spirit, soul, and body—reflects an overall priority order for life. In view of this, we are convinced that the place to begin confronting cancer is at the spiritual level.

This starts, as Angela, Jessica, Candy, Doc, and others discovered, with personal faith in Jesus Christ. The reason is obvious. The entire human race has been infected in the spiritual realm with a cancer-like disease called sin. Like cancer, sin may at times be difficult, if not impossible, to spot. However, also like cancer in the physical realm, sin runs its course in the spiritual realm—often with serious emotional and physical consequences. And its ultimate product is death (James 1:15).

The only way to reverse this consequence is through the provision of Jesus Christ, who died as God's perfect sacrifice to take away sin. Covering sin up, countering its effects with religious activities, or pretending it doesn't exist simply will not work, no more than cosmetics or physical exercise can stop cancer in its tracks. Just as radical action is necessary to deal with the catastrophic consequences of cancer, so it is with sin.

God's provision of His Son Jesus Christ, who died and arose to provide everlasting life to be received as a free gift, is the only answer for mankind's sin problem. We are convinced that the ultimate key to successfully coping with cancer, or any of life's other traumas, comes from the resources we receive from God when we trust His Son as our Savior.

Angela summed it up so well when she said, "I just don't know how I would have handled this apart from my faith. There were plenty of people who could encourage me. I had the best medical care. That was good, up to a point. But ultimately, my relationship with the Lord provided me with the resources I needed."

Remembering the difficult days of Doc's battle with pancreatic cancer, Shannon observed, "We had plenty of help and encouragement from friends. We had the best knowledge we could get our hands on. But the most important factor was our faith. We couldn't even *begin* to give each other the strength we needed for those horrible experiences. Our faith in the Lord was what ultimately brought us through."

Ron took the principle of faith a step beyond salvation as he reflected on God's sovereign care in life's circumstances. "Dianna and I had to remember that God's goodness and sovereignty guaranteed that, whatever happened with Jessica, we would not allow ourselves to become bitter toward Him. He's far too good to let anything happen to us that does not ultimately have some positive purpose, even though the event may not be good in itself. And He's much too powerful not to be in absolute control. Even though many people use it tritely as a biblical Band-Aid, I'm convinced that the truth of Romans 8:28 is a key part of what sustained us. We know that God works all things together for good to those who love Him, to those who are called according to His purpose. We know He loves Jessica. We know He loves us. And we simply trust Him."

Candy emphasized the one-day-at-a-time approach to faith and life. Now actively involved in helping others overcome physical disfiguration by emphasizing healthy personal appearance rather than beauty, she is quick to point out, "I've learned to gain strength for each day, one day at a time. I can't take care of tomorrow or the day after—or next month or three years down the road. I know there's always the possibility that the cancer will come back. But if I trust God and take care of my areas of responsibility—getting regular checkups, eating right, things like that—then I can take each day a step at a time, knowing my walk with the Lord will bring me through."

Sustained by Hope

Hope is an all-important dimension that originates in the spiritual realm but impacts us in the emotional. For Cliff, hope played a key role throughout the darkest days of his battle with colon cancer. Years later, when he was diagnosed with liver cancer, he continued to rely on hope to sustain him. "I've studied the Scriptures on hope quite extensively. Hope is not simply some self-generated, positive feeling about the future. It's a response of certainty to what God has told us He has done—and is doing. And it's the key factor to keep us going, no matter how difficult the battle with an enemy like cancer may become."

Eminent psychiatrist Karl Menninger identifies hope as perhaps the key factor in any patient's recovery from disease.[5] Attacking the futility of what he terms "hopeless physicians providing over hopeless patients," Menninger calls upon the medical community to communicate hope and on patients to exercise hope.

It is our conviction that biblical hope is the only kind that will work in the desperate setting of a diagnosis like cancer. The essence of such hope is a positive expectation regarding the future based on a propositional reality from the past—the reality of the resurrection of Jesus Christ.[6] Christian hope is firmly rooted in the ultimate victory over sin and death to which

Paul pointed in 1 Corinthians 15—the resurrection. Because Christ overcame sin and death, we can experience hope. This hope has two implications for when cancer comes.

First, we don't give up. We do not quit. As Casey was so quick to put it, "Even though we knew we were losing Debbie, when we sensed her death was going to occur, we still never lost hope. We never gave up on God. In fact, the day she died, I was still praying that if God were pleased, He would work a miracle to bring her through."

The second implication is what Casey hinted at when he used the words "if God were pleased." Genuine biblical hope recognizes that its ultimate focus is not in this life but on that which is to come. The apostle Paul points out this vital balance in 2 Corinthians 4:16–18, reminding his readers that we must not give up, even in great adversity: "Even though our outward man is perishing, yet the inward man is being renewed day by day." This statement from the apostle is loaded with practical significance for the cancer patient. The outward evidences of impending death may increase with each passing day. Yet the inward strength provided by spiritual renewal is abundantly sufficient: "Our light affliction, which is but for a moment, is working for us a far more exceeding and eternal weight of glory, while we look not at the things which are seen, but at the things which are not seen. For the things which are seen are temporary, but the things which are not seen are eternal."

The essence of what Paul is saying is that hope allows us to cope day by day with life's drastic adversities, not focusing on present suffering, trauma, or discouraging circumstances, but on the ultimate reality: a future glory in heaven based on the resurrection through which Christ overcame the final enemy, death.

Such hope sustained Betty and Jimmy (chapter 11) during the loss of so many brothers and sisters. "It's hard to lose those who are close to you—especially when you know it could happen to you," Jimmy noted. "But through it all we kept our hope and confidence focused on God." Betty said, "Each time, we just sensed we had to draw a little closer to God. Let Him help us work through our grief, and keep going. He gave us the support we needed as we kept trusting Him. That also helped us realize how we needed to start supporting each other more."

Supported by Others

Whether in the formal setting of a cancer support group, the warmth of a loving family environment, or through gathering regularly with concerned Christian friends from a local church, that kind of emotional support is absolutely crucial.

Doc and Shannon experienced it from their friends at Rapha as well as others in the Christian community. "So many people came, helped, called and shared with us," Shannon recalled. "Especially that small core of supportive people we came to count on."

For Casey and Debbie, and for Jessica and her parents, the local church family proved to be a source of essential emotional resources and support. "They were there for us," Casey remembered. "Our pastor, our Sunday school class, other close friends—they called, they came to the hospital, they brought food, they did all kinds of tangible things. It was like a whole mass of loving people just put their arms around Debbie and me, and loved us through that terrible time."

Ron recalled "hundreds of people staying up late at night, praying, gathering at the church, coming by the hospital. They were family to us. They accepted us. They didn't expect us to perform. They just let us know they loved us."

Candy was quick to point out the benefits of the cancer support group she and her husband attended. "We're not attending now, but when we first came through all the surgeries and the diagnosis, things were really tough for the two of us. Getting into that cancer support group was the best thing we could have done."

Shannon recalls, "That close core of friends allowed Jim and me to share our fears, our anger, the reality of our struggles. And struggle we did—but they accepted us in low times as well as high. We desperately needed that. I think every person with cancer, and every family member, has to have that kind of human support."

For Tom, his administrative assistant, Judith, provided a key support role, both during his cancer treatment and in taking care of his business. "I was extremely reluctant to even get into the treatment program, because I had so much to do with my business. But Judith assured me that she and the rest of the team would take care of things. And since I had almost nobody in the way of family I could turn to, she and her two sons were like family to me. Especially when I was sickest. They provided meals, helped with chores around the house, all those kinds of things."

Cliff especially appreciated the support of the excellent medical care he received. "I tend to be a bit of a skeptical person, but my personal physician, my surgeon, my radiologist, and my oncologist all took the time to explain things to me. They let me know what was going on. They were honest with me. I felt they gave me an extra measure of personal attention, along with excellent professional care."

Phyllis recalled how her doctor helped her face reality. "I didn't want to even consider the possibility that I had cancer. I was in so much denial, I was close to refusing to take the steps to get the medical care I needed. Having a doctor who took the time to explain things to me, to communicate clearly just how serious things were, but who also let me know that there was hope for me as long as I made sure to get the right treatment— that was crucial."

Choices for the Patient

When you have been diagnosed with cancer, sometimes you feel that you no longer have choices. There is a sense in which one choice has been eliminated. You can no longer choose *not* to have cancer. You cannot choose to have cancer become a *non*factor in your life. However, there are still choices available—choices in the physical and medical, choices in the emotional and relational, and choices in the spiritual realm. Making the right choices can help you cope when cancer comes.

In the physical realm, your first logical choice is to gather as much information as possible to help you understand cancer. Choose to seek out the best medical care, including second and third opinions when appropriate. But as you learn to rely on that care, choose to take personal responsibility for getting the ongoing medical care you need. Choose to maintain a healthy routine to the degree possible, including proper diet and cutting down on carcinogens. And choose to take personal responsibility without ignoring the balance of accepting help and encouragement from family, friends, and others.

Emotionally, the most important choice is to share your feelings, fears, anger, and other emotions openly and appropriately with family, friends, your minister, and—if needed—a counselor. We also encourage cancer patients to choose to take their minds off themselves, to focus on others and their pain. Another important choice is to continue gathering information without becoming obsessed with cancer information and related concerns. Although cancer is a major part of life, it is not the sum total of life, even for the most seriously ill cancer patient. Focusing on things in your life other than cancer and focusing on others is not only emotionally healthy and biblically appropriate, it is essential.

Finally, in the spiritual realm, we encourage you to choose hope—not a blind hope that ignores the possibility that the cancer treatment you are pursuing may not be successful, but one that recognizes that, for the believer, "to live is Christ, and to die is gain" (Philippians 1:21). We also encourage the choice of refusing to allow bitterness to infect your life. Choose to practice the therapy of thankfulness, while looking for the good God may bring into even the worst of circumstances. Sure, there are many things that are not desirable, that are extremely frustrating, that produce pain, anger, and fear. But we encourage a strong focus on personal faith, meditating on Scripture, personal and individual worship, and prayer—the disciplines of godly living, including worshiping with God's people at church when health permits.

Some of these choices may seem easy. Others may appear difficult beyond imagination. Yet making the right choices is not optional, it is essential for coping with cancer. There's a simple reason: Having cancer is like warfare. Those who find themselves in the middle of a war simply cannot choose to ignore it. It doesn't go away. However, when those who have cancer and those who are close to them choose to engage in combat against cancer when it comes, the war becomes winnable. The choice is yours.

NOTES

CHAPTER 1

1. Mark Rennaker, M.D., *Understanding Cancer*, 3d ed. (Menlo Park, Calif.: Bull, 1988), 2.
2. Ibid., 260.

CHAPTER 2

1. *Journal of Psychology and Christianity* 2, no. 1 (Spring 1983), 12.
2. Rennaker, *Understanding Cancer*, 3.
3. Ibid, 4.

CHAPTER 3

1. Morton T. Kelsey, *Healing and Christianity* (New York: Harper & Row, 1963), 54.
2. Rennaker, *Understanding Cancer*, 9.
3. Ibid.
4. See Merrill F. Unger, *The New Unger's Bible Dictionary* (Chicago: Moody, 1988), 305–8; J. D. Douglas and N. Hillyer, *The Illustrated Bible Dictionary* (Wheaton: Tyndale, 1980), 616–20.
5. Frank Minirth and Ike Minirth, with Georgia Minirth Beech and Mary Alice Minirth, *Beating the Odds: Overcoming Life's Trials* (Grand Rapids: Baker, 1987), 105-17.
6. Ibid., 116.
7. Dialogue taken from the Public Television special "Shadow Lands," quoted in Don Hawkins, *Never Give Up* (San Bernadino, Calif.: Here's Life, 1992), 103.

CHAPTER 4

1. Rennaker, *Understanding Cancer*, 20.

2. Malin Dollinger, M.D., Ernest Rosenbaum, M.D., and Greg Cable, *Everyone's Guide to Cancer Therapy* (New York: Andrews & McNeel, 1991), 11.

3. Sir Richard Doll and Richard Peto, "The Causes of Cancer," *Journal of the National Cancer Institute* 66, no. 6 (June 1981).

4. Rennaker, *Understanding Cancer*, 83.

CHAPTER 5

1. Dollinger, Rosenbaum, and Cable, *Everyone's Guide to Cancer Therapy*, 5.

CHAPTER 6

1. W. E. Vine, *An Expository Dictionary of New Testament Words* (Old Tappan, N.J.: Revell, 1940), 168.

2. Wendy S. Harpham, *Diagnosis: Cancer* (New York: W. W. Norton, 1992), xi.

3. Harold Kaplan, M.D., and Benjamin Sadock, M.D., *Synopsis of Psychiatry*, 5th ed. (Baltimore: Williams & Wilkins, 1988).

4. Donald D. Nichols, M.D., "The Cancer Experience & Kübler-Ross's Stages of Dying," *Journal of Psychology & Christianity* 2, no. 1 (Spring 1983), 15. Even though Kübler-Ross was a New Age spokesperson (William Watson, *A Concise Dictionary of Cults and Religion* [Chicago: Moody, 1991]), her stages of grief have gained widespread acceptance because they are based on universal human experience rather than on her personal religious views.

CHAPTER 7

1. John F. Walvoord and Roy B. Zuck, eds., *Bible Knowledge Commentary* (Wheaton, Ill.: Victor, 1983), 583.

2. Gary Smalley and Al Janssen, *Joy That Lasts* (Grand Rapids: Zondervan, 1986), 121.

3. Frank Gaebelein, ed., *Expositor's Bible Commentary* (Grand Rapids: Zondervan, 1981), 12:204.

4. Walvoord and Zuck, eds., *Bible Knowledge Commentary*, 835.

CHAPTER 9

1. Renneker, *Understanding Cancer*, 178.

2. Lawrence J. Crabb and Dan B. Allender, *Encouragement: Key to Caring* (Grand Rapids: Zondervan, 1984), 73–78.

CHAPTER 10

1. *People* magazine, 2 November 1992, 115.

2. *Sports Illustrated*, 25 January 1993, 48.

3. Renneker, *Understanding Cancer*, 4.

4. Marion Morra and Eve Pots, *Choices: Realistic Alternatives in Cancer Treatment*, rev. ed., (New York: Avon, 1987), 1.

5. *USA Today*, 25 November 1992.

6. Harold Ivan Smith, *Positively Single* (Wheaton, Ill.: Victor, 1986), 129.

7. Phillip Yancey, "Death Whispers," *Christianity Today* 32, no. 9 (13 May 1988), 25.

8. Elizabeth Elliot, *Passion and Purity* (Old Tappan, N.J.: Revell, 1984), 80.

9. *Dallas Morning News*, Sunday, 6 September 1992.

10. Robert S. McGee, *Dealing with Pain* (Houston: Rapha, 1988), 2.

11. Ibid., 7. For additional resources on pain and suffering, see C. S. Lewis, *The Problem of Pain* (New York: McMillan, 1962); Phillip Yancey, *Where Is God When It Hurts?* (Grand Rapids: Zondervan, 1977).

12. Elizabeth Stark, "Breaking the Pain Habit," *Psychology Today* (May 1985), 31–36.

13. Elizabeth Kübler-Ross, *On Death and Dying* (New York: Macmillan, 1969). Even though Kübler-Ross was a New Age spokesperson (William Watson, *A Concise Dictionary of Cults and Religion* [Chicago: Moody, 1991]), her stages of grief have gained widespread acceptance because they are based on universal human experience rather than on her personal religious views.

14. Billy Graham, *Facing Death and the Life After* (Waco, Tex.: Word, 1987), 164.

15. Kübler-Ross, *On Death and Dying*.

CHAPTER 11

1. Renneker, *Understanding Cancer*, 7.

2. Jeff Lyon, "Herbal arsenal: Garlic and its cousins may be the best weapons yet in preventing disease," Tempo section, *Chicago Tribune*, 20 December 1992; *Dallas Morning News*, 1 March 1993, 3–4C.

3. Ibid.

4. Ibid.

Glossary

adenocarcinoma (sometimes referred to as adenoma) cancer originating in glandular tissue, such as breast, lung, thyroid, or pancreas.

adjuvant chemotherapy chemotherapy given when there is no test evidence of leftover cancer cells but there is reason for concern over the presence of undetected cancer cells in the body; its purpose is to decrease the chance of a recurrence.

aerobic system an oxygen-dependent respiratory system; human and animal cells operate on an aerobic system, that is, they are dependent on oxygen for life.

agglutination collection of the cells distributed in a fluid into clumps.

AIDS (acquired immunodeficiency syndrome) a viral infection-caused disease that weakens the immune system by killing a key "helper" cell (T4), which causes characteristic symptoms and often manifests in Kaposi's sarcoma.

ALG (antilymphocyte globulin) powerful immunosuppressive agent made to work against the lymphocytes or lymphocyte globulins.

alpha particles high-energy particles dispensing their energy in a very limited range within tissues, but highly destructive of the tissues they encounter.

amino acids organic compounds, the building blocks for proteins; some of these acids are essential for life.

anaplastic cancerous; anaplastic cells have reverted to a primitive or undifferentiated form.

anaploid cells cells containing an abnormal number of chromosomes; considered to be cancerous.

anemia low blood count, low red blood cells or hemoglobin, caused by blood loss, blood destruction in the vessels, or an impaired ability to manufacture new blood.

angiogram an X ray of blood vessels, taken after the injection of dye.

antibiotic a substance produced by living organisms, such as bacteria or moles, that can destroy other bacteria; the most familiar example is penicillin; certain antibiotics have been shown to be effective anticancer agents.

antibody substance manufactured by cells to fight invading antigens.

antigen a foreign substance, such as the antigen of a virus, invading a cell, which leads to the formation of antibodies.

ATP (adenosine triphosphate) a nucleotide compound occurring in all cells, an energy source for cellular function.

axilla the small hollow beneath the arm, where it joins the shoulder; also called the armpit.

axillary lymph nodes lymph nodes located in the axilla.

bacteria single-celled organisms; many are infectious.

barium enema the use of barium sulfate introduced into the intestinal tract by an enema to allow X-ray exam of the lower bowel (colon and rectum).

barium swallow an X ray of the pharynx, or throat, and esophagus; a barium-containing liquid is swallowed and X rays are taken during the swallowing process to show the contractions of the esophagus and outline the inner surface of the esophagus and pharynx.

basal cell carcinoma the most common type of skin cancer; forms in the lower-most layer of the skin, grows slowly, and seldom spreads; easily detected, it is readily cured when treated properly.

benign tumor   an abnormal growth or swelling that is not a cancer; cannot spread to other parts of the body and is usually harmless, but can sometimes cause problems because of its location.

biochemical markers   proteins that are detected in abnormal amounts in the blood or at the site of a cancer; used to diagnose and follow certain cancers; even with today's advanced technology, only certain cancers have biochemical markers that are useful in patient care.

biological therapy   treatment by stimulation of the body's immune defense system, often referred to as immunotherapy.

biopsy   the removal of a small portion of tissue from the body of a living person for examination under the microscope.

blood count   an examination of the blood to count the number of white and red cells and platelets.

bone marrow   the soft substance in the center of bones, the place where blood is made.

bone marrow biopsy   procedure to obtain a sample of bone marrow for analysis, usually obtained from the hip or breast bone; a local anesthetic is used, then a special needle is placed into the bone and a sample of the marrow withdrawn.

bone scan   a picture of all the bones in the body using a small amount of injected radioactive substance; abnormalities show up as areas of increased or decreased radioactivity.

breast self-examination   simple procedure to examine the breasts thoroughly, recommended for all women as a monthly procedure between regular physician checkups.

cachexia   severe generalized weakness, malnutrition, and emaciation; frequently found in the end stages of terminal cancer, the destructive result of tumor growth on the human body.

cancer   the general term for a large number of diseases characterized by abnormal and uncontrolled growth and spread of cells; the mass, or tumor, can invade and destroy surrounding normal tissues; cancer cells can spread through the blood or lymph system to start new cancers in other parts of the body.

carcinogen   an agent—chemical, viral, or irradiating—capable of inducing cancer.

carcinoma a form of cancer that begins in the tissues that cover or line certain organs or ducts, such as the intestines, uterus, lung, breast, or skin.

carcinoma in situ a stage in the growth of a cancer when it is still confined to the tissue in which it started.

CAT scan (computerized axial tomography), also referred to as CT scan (computerized tomography) this sophisticated X-ray procedure shows cross-sectional views of the area in pictures, using computer processing; the test frequently necessitates taking contrast material by mouth or injecting dye into a vein.

chemotherapy treatment with anticancer drugs.

chromosomes minute structures in the cell nucleus made up of genes; chromosomes are the carriers of heredity.

clinical pertaining to the study and treatment of disease in human beings by direct observation, as distinguished from laboratory research.

colonoscopy technique used to visually examine the entire large bowel by means of a lighted, flexible tube.

colostomy a surgical procedure that creates an artificial opening from the colon through the abdominal wall to permit the elimination of waste into an external pouch.

combination therapy use of two or more modes of treatment, such as surgery, radiotherapy, chemotherapy, or immunotherapy, in combination (alternately or together) in order to achieve optimum results against cancer.

CSF (colony stimulating factor) a substance produced by the healthy body to regulate the number and function of blood cells; CSFs can be produced artificially, and studies are underway to determine how they can help cancer patients tolerate cancer therapy and fight cancer; may help overcome some of the most serious complications to cancer therapy, including susceptibility to bacterial infection and risk of bleeding.

cure when doctors talk of a cancer cure, they usually mean there is no detectable sign of cancer, and the person has the same life expectancy as if he or she never had cancer; sometimes the word *cure* is used when there is no evidence of cancer for at least five years, although the cure time for every cancer is different.

cyst sac containing fluid and/or solid material; usually benign but can be malignant.

cystogram an X ray of the urinary bladder after dye has been introduced into the bladder through a catheter.

cytology the science that deals with the study of living cells; cells scraped off or sloughed off from organs, such as the uterus, bladder, lungs, or stomach, are examined under the microscope for early signs of abnormality; the Pap test for cervical cancer is an example of cytology.

DES (diethylstilbestrol) synthetic compound, often linked to adenocarcinoma of the vagina.

diagnosis identifying or naming a disease by its signs, symptoms, course, and laboratory findings.

differentiation the development of form and function in a cell or tissue.

diverticulosis a common condition affecting the intestines, where small pockets, or diverticula, develop as a result of weak points in the bowel wall; when these pockets become infected, the condition is called diverticulitis.

DNA (deoxyribonucleic acid) the informational macromolecules of the cell nucleus, wound together in a double helix form.

dysplasia disturbance in the usual, orderly organization of cells and tissues, often on epidermic and mucosal surfaces; frequently dysplasia is part of the developmental phase of many neoplasms.

edema the presence of large amounts of fluid in the intercellular space of the body.

electron microscopy a technique for visualizing material through a microscope using beams of electrons, or negative electrical units, instead of light beams; this process permits clearer magnification than is possible with an ordinary microscope.

endocrine glands glands secreting internally into the blood or lymph system.

endogenous originating or developing with the organism.

endoscopy the use of a scope to examine a body cavity.

epidemiologist a health professional/statistician who detects disease patterns through the evaluation of data related to the incidence and prevalence of the disease.

epidemiology the study of incidence, distribution, environmental causes, and control of a disease within a population.

esophageal speech an acquired technique by which those who have had their voice boxes surgically removed are taught to speak again by swallowing, then expelling air through the mouth from the esophagus.

etiology the study of the causes of disease.

excision surgical removal of a diseased part of the body, including cancerous growths.

exogenous originating or developing outside of an organism.

fiber the structural component of plant cell walls that is not digested by human gastrointestinal enzymes; fiber can be soluble or insoluble.

fine-needle aspiration using a needle to biopsy a tumor through the skin.

gallium scan a picture of the body taken by scanner using a small amount of radioactive substance to show areas of inflammation or dividing cells.

gamete one of two cells, male and female, whose union is necessary to initiate the development of a new individual by means of sexual reproduction.

gamma rays the electromagnetic radiation of short wavelength, emitted by the nucleus of an atom during a nuclear reaction.

Gemcitabine an investigational form of chemotherapy.

genes units of hereditary material grouped into chromosomes, made up of DNA.

genetic code a sequence of organic compounds in DNA, which carry the hereditary message for protein synthesis.

guaiac test a chemical test used to detect occult, or hidden, blood in the stool; stool specimens are placed on special guaiac-treated paper slides that are checked by a doctor or lab technician; the test is ideal for screening programs for colorectal cancer, since the specimen can be prepared at home.

HIV (human immunodeficiency virus) the AIDS virus, also called HTLV-3.

Hodgkin's disease a cancer of the lymphatic system.

homeostasis the essential stability of an organism.

hormonal therapy the use of hormones to treat cancer.

hormone status the hormone status of an individual's cancer is determined by sophisticated tests done on a piece of the tumor; those tests indicate which hormones may affect the cancer cells; hormone status can only be determined for a few types of cancer.

hyperplasia the abnormal multiplication of cells in a tissue.

hyperthermia abnormally high body temperature, especially when induced for therapeutic reasons.

hysterectomy a surgical procedure for removing the uterus, frequently combined with removal of the ovaries, or oophorectomy.

ileostomy a surgical procedure to form an artificial opening of the small intestine through the abdominal wall for the elimination of body waste.

immune system white blood cells and antibodies that protect the body by attacking foreign substances.

immunology the science of immunity or the study of the mechanisms by which the host reacts to foreign substances in its environment to resist disease, infection, or poison.

immunosuppression suppression of the body's immune responses; certain chemicals initiate immunosuppression.

immunotherapy treatment of disease by stimulating the body's own defense mechanisms against the disease.

in situ confined to a small site of origin, frequently referred to as cancer in situ.

induction therapy the initial treatment to eliminate or control cancer.

initiation (of cancer process) the silent beginning of the cancer process.

initiator an agent that initiates the growth of a cancer.

interferons   special proteins made by cells to fight virus infections; have been found to have certain anticancer properties.

interleukin   a chemical produced as part of an immune response.

investigational therapy   cancer treatments undergoing clinical testing to determine their safety, efficacy, and benefit.

IVP (intravenous pyleogram)   an X ray of the kidneys, taken after a dye is injected into the vein, to show whether kidney function is normal.

Kaposi's sarcoma   before the AIDS epidemic, classic Kaposi's sarcoma was known as a slow-growing cancer of the skin of the legs; Kaposi's sarcoma in the AIDS patient involves widespread cancer of the skin and frequently spreads to the lymph nodes, gastrointestinal tract, and lungs.

laryngectomy   a surgical procedure to remove the larynx, or voice box.

laser (light amplification by stimulated emission of radiation)   a narrow, intensely powerful beam of radiation.

lesion   any abnormal change in tissue due to disease or injury.

leukemia   cancer of the blood-forming tissues, including bone marrow, lymph nodes, or spleen, characterized by the overproduction of white blood cells.

leukoplakia   whitish, thickened patch of the epithelium, sometimes a forerunner to cancer.

leukocytosis   proliferation of leukocyte-forming tissue, the basis of leukemia.

linear accelerator   a machine producing high-energy radiation.

liver-spleen scan   a picture taken of the liver and spleen using a small amount of radioactive tracer injected into the vein.

living will   a written document that outlines how much you want doctors to do to prolong your life, with medicines and machines, if you become critically ill with little hope of recovery.

localized   limited to the site of origin, with no evidence of spread.

lumbar puncture   also known as a spinal tap; after a local anesthetic is used, a needle is inserted into the spine to draw a sample of spinal fluid.

lymph fluid   a clear fluid that circulates through the body, containing white blood cells, antibodies, and nourishing substances; lymph fluid is filtered in the lymph nodes, then added to the bloodstream.

lymph nodes   rounded, bean-shaped organs that make some of the white blood cells, such as lymphocytes and monocytes, then filter the lymph fluid before it enters the blood; the human body contains thousands of them, ranging from pinhead size to the approximate size of an olive; the most obvious ones are in the neck, armpit, and groin; cancer frequently spreads to the lymph nodes.

lymphangiogram   an X ray of the lymph nodes in the pelvis and abdomen area; dye is injected into the veins in the feet, and the X rays are taken a few minutes later.

lymphatic system   a circulation system, like the blood system, that carries lymph fluid, a colorless fluid carrying infection-fighting cells, throughout the body; the lymph organs include the lymph nodes, spleen, and thymus.

lymphoblastoma   a cancer of the lymphatic system.

lymphoma   a cancer of the lymphatic system.

lymphosarcoma   a cancer of lymphatic system. (*See* lymphoma)

malignant   cancerous; a malignant tumor is an aggressive, abnormal tissue growth that tends to destroy the host by direct spread or metastasis.

mammography   low-dose X-ray technique for studying the structure of breast tissue to detect any abnormality or possibility of breast cancer at the earliest possible stage.

mastectomy   surgical removal of a cancerous breast to prevent the spread of the disease; simple mastectomy refers to the removal of the entire breast; radical mastectomy also involves removing underlying muscle tissue and lymph nodes in the armpit.

melanoma   a pigmented, highly malignant form of cancer of the skin; tumor may vary in color from almost white to nearly black.

mesothelioma   a tumor formed from cells that line the inside of the body; malignant mesothelioma is increasingly common, but still rare; cancer associated with exposure to asbestos.

metabolism   all the physical and chemical processes in living organisms necessary to maintain life.

metastasis (pl., metastases)   cancer cells that have spread from their original site, usually by blood or lymph streams, creating secondary tumor centers at a distance from the original tumor.

metastasize   to spread.

mitosis   cell division.

modality   a method of treating a disease such as cancer; surgery and chemotherapy are examples of treatment modalities.

monoclonal antibody therapy   a new technique being investigated for treating cancer, involving specific antibodies produced in the laboratory using recombinant DNA technology; these antibodies will react specifically with cancer cells.

morbidity   conditions of being diseased.

MRI or MRI scan (magnetic resonance imaging)   diagnostic imaging technique that uses a magnetic field and radio waves instead of X rays; the pictures obtained are quite detailed; the procedure is similar to a CAT scan, but does not expose the patient to radiation.

multiple myeloma   cancer of the plasma cells and the bone marrow.

mutant   the result of a mutation or change.

mutation   change in a cell that is permanent and transmissible to offspring cells.

myelogram   an X-ray test of the spinal cord, after dye has been injected through a spinal tap into the spinal fluid; frequently a CT scan is done after the myelogram.

necrosis   death of tissue.

neoplasia   the process of new growth, a term used commonly for cancer formation.

neoplasm tumor; an abnormal growth of cells or tissues; may be benign or malignant, but is frequently used to describe a cancerous growth.

neoplastic transformation the change from normal growth to abnormal growth, such as a tumor.

nodule a lump or tumor; may be malignant or benign.

non-Hodgkin's lymphoma a type of cancer of the lymphatic system.

obstructive edema swelling of the limbs due to choking of the lymphatic channels by cancer cells.

oncogenesis the development of a tumor or growth.

oncogenic leading to the development of a tumor or growth.

oncologist a physician who specializes in cancer diagnosis and treatment.

oncology the study of cancer, which has become a specialty branch of modern medicine.

ostomy a surgical procedure to create an opening in the skin to allow connection to an internal organ for drainage.

palliative treatment providing relief from symptoms of a disease but not directly curing the disease; alleviating pain.

palpation the application of the fingers to the body for the purpose of diagnosis.

Pap test procedure developed by the late Dr. George Papanicolaou to microscopically examine cells from vaginal secretions in order to detect cancer of the cervix.

pathologist doctor who specializes in diagnosing disease; frequently performs autopsies and examines urine, blood, tissues removed for biopsies, etc., using microscopic and other technologies.

pathology the science that studies the nature, cause, and development of disease through examination of bodily tissues and fluids.

platelet small circular or oval disc present in the blood, which is necessary for the blood to clot in order to stop bleeding.

pneumonectomy   surgical procedure for removing an entire lung.

polyp   an overgrowth of tissue projecting into a body cavity, such as the lining of the colon, the nasal passage, or the surface of vocal cords.

polyposis   the development of multiple polyps in an organ or structure.

primary lesion   place where the cancer first started.

procto   short for proctosigmoidoscopy, an examination of the first ten inches of the rectum and colon with a hollow, lighted tube.

prognosis   the prospect of a disease; prediction of how well the patient will do.

promoter   an agent that causes a cancer to grow, or grow more rapidly, after the cancer has been initiated; promotion includes the intermediate stages of cancer growth, in which the cell is altered by extraneous factors, either from within the patient or from the environment.

prophase   followed by metaphase, anaphase, and telophase; the four main phases of cell division.

protocol   description of the treatment steps, the "recipe" for cancer therapy.

quackery   the practice of using untested or unproven methods of treatment for a disease; alleged recoveries cannot be validated or equaled in subsequent tests under controlled situations.

rad   a measure of the amount of any ionizing radiation that is absorbed by tissue.

radiation sickness   illness sometimes caused by radiation therapy, characterized by nausea, lack of appetite, vomiting, and diarrhea.

radiation therapy (or radiotherapy)   treatment of cancer with radiant energy of extremely short wavelengths in order to damage or kill cancer cells; radioactive substances such as cobalt 60, radium, gallium, and cesium 27 are often used to produce gamma rays; betatrons and linear accelerators are used to produce X rays.

radiotherapist physician who specializes in the treatment of disease by means of radiation therapy.

receptor expression how specific receptors are found on the surface of a cancer cell, and how effective they are at doing their jobs; determination of receptor expression may one day lead to the development of cancer therapy that only kills cancer cells, while leaving normal cells alone.

receptors proteins on the surface of all cells that bind with available complimentary proteins; some receptors are found only on normal cells, some are found on both normal and cancer cells, and some only on cancer cells; sophisticated tests can now identify the presence of some receptors.

recurrence reappearance of the same cancer after a period when there was no evidence of cancer.

regional involvement when cancer has spread from its original site to a nearby area (metastasis).

regression when a disease or symptom subsides.

remission complete or partial disappearance of signs and symptoms of a disease; partial or complete shrinkage of a cancer; also refers to the period in which a disease is under control.

replication the self-copying processes of cell division; the transcription and translation of the genetic coding from one cell generation to the next.

residual disease remaining cancer or tumor.

sarcoma cancer of the soft or connective tissue, such as bones, cartilage, muscles, nerves, or tendons.

sigmoidoscopy visual inspection of the lower portion of the large bowel (the sigmoid colon).

sputum test, or sputum cytology a study of the cells from the lungs contained in material coughed up in the sputum.

staging determining the extent of growth of a cancer so treatment results can be compared and a prognosis offered.

T-cells lymphocyte responsible for cell-mediated immunity; the "T" stands for "thymus dependent."

tissue a collection of similar cells; there are four basic tissues in the body: epithelial, connective, muscle, and nerve.

TNF (tumor necrosis factor) proteins that are released by certain white blood cells in response to bacterial infection; laboratory tests have shown these proteins to be lethal to some cancer cells; studies are underway to evaluate the safety and efficacy of TNFs in cancer patients.

tolerance the state of acceptance of an antigen by the cell, or response of an organism to a drug.

tomograms cross-sectional X rays.

toxicologist a scientist who investigates, in a laboratory, the association between exposure to a chemical and its biological effect.

transformation conversion of a normal cell into an abnormal cell, usually a cancer cell, because of the influence of radiation, chemicals, or viruses.

tumor an abnormal swelling or enlargement; mass of tissue, either benign or malignant.

ultrasound a fast, noninvasive, and safe technique that uses sound waves to create pictures of the inside of the body.

upper GI an X ray of the stomach, taken after a contrast-containing solution is swallowed.

virus a molecular composite consisting of an inner nucleic acid core and an outer protein coat; viruses are parasitic, that is, they need to live in a cell to reproduce.

X ray also referred to as plane radiography, pictures taken using low-dose exposure to radiant energy of extremely short wavelength; frequently used in the diagnosis and treatment of cancer.